"Lia Schorr has unmasked the mysteries of the skin throughout her years of research and practical application. Her words of skin-care wisdom are an inspiration to anyone interested in good, clean, healthy skin."

—Maggie Mulhern
Beauty and Fashion
Editor
Modern Salon magazine

"My fifteen years' experience as a beauty writer has taken me all over the world to review the top beauty services and products, but when I choose where to go for my own personal beauty needs, it is always to Lia Schorr's New York salon. Amidst all the outlandish trends, the wild promises and extravagant fees of the beauty field, Lia's approach to helping women make the most of their looks stands out as being sane, sensible, intelligent and reasonable. A working mother herself, she is aware of and sensitive to the important role lifestyle plays in a good beauty routine for contemporary, busy women. Lia Schorr is the thinking woman's beauty expert—a beauty herself, she generously shares all her knowledge and wisdom with all who come into contact with her."

—Susan Duff
Beauty Author
*Mademoiselle, Harper's
Bazaar, Cosmopolitan*
magazines

"Lia Schorr knows her business—she is a constant source of skin information. Viva Lia!!"

—Linda Staci
Health and Beauty
Editor
Elle

"Lia Schorr is a truly creative skin-care practitioner. She deals with the skin in context, relating it to the totality of biology, diet, emotion, environment and season. I have found her tips, treatments and suggestions to be often original and always practical."

—Joanna Brown
Contributing Editor
Personal Grooming/
Fashion
VIS a VIS (Airline/
Travel Magazine)

"As a performer, my appearance counts. Lia Schorr's advice has saved my skin from the heat of stage lights, the stress from travel and the dry, overheated air of recording studios. I'm one of her true fans."

—Melba Moore
Singer/Dancer/
Entertainer

"The TV cameras exaggerate every spot or line on your skin. Lia Schorr helps keep my complexion looking perfectly smooth—even under television's bright glare!"

—Eileen Fulton
Actress
Lisa on "As the World Turns"

"Lia Schorr has established herself as a prominent figure in the skin-care industry. Utilizing the mediums of *Better Nutrition* and *Today's Living* magazines, she has communicated her helpful advice to an audience concerned not only with internal health, but also with external appearance via healthy habits and a natural skin-care regimen. In this day and age of self-help information, Lia's practical, concise style puts her in the forefront."

—Patti Seikus
Better Nutrition and
Today's Living
magazines

"As a dermatologist, I sometimes hesitate to send a woman to a skin-care salon, but Lia Schorr is a cut above the rest. Her advice is practical and knowledgeable, and equally important, she knows when a skin problem belongs in a doctor's hands."

—John F. Romano, M.D.
Dermatologist

"Lia Schorr's approach to skin care goes beyond cremes and lotions. Put yourself in Lia's hands and you will learn good skin care habits that will reward you with a lifetime of beautiful skin."

—Carol Straley
Beauty Editor
Parents Magazine

"Lia Schorr raises the science of skin care to a fine art. *Lia Schorr's Seasonal Skin Care* glows with the wisdom and clarity of this world-reknowned expert. No skin should be without it."

—Paulette Weiss
Beauty Editor
Where Magazine

"Take it from me—just one visit to Lia Schorr is a total panacea. Not only does your skin look and feel wonderful, you transcend into a state of total relaxation! That's why this book is a must for people who cannot visit Lia's salon in New York."

—Patricia Ford
Editor-in-Chief
Beauty Handbook

"Lia Schorr has been a source of quality information and time saving hints for the business woman who needs a beauty regime that will keep her radiant all day."

—Jane Heiles Gyulavary
Fashion and Beauty
Editor
Working Woman

"Ms. Lia Schorr, contributing writer to *Les Nouvelles Esthétiques* American Edition since its birth, is one of the leading authorities in the field of esthetics. To *Les Nouvelles Esthétiques* American Edition she is an important source of knowledge, expressed in a wealth of up-to-date articles which enlighten without failing to entertain her readers. Her innovative, creative ideas are presented in a practical, easy-to-follow approach to skin care."

—Elke Zimmermann
Managing Editor
*Les Nouvelles
Esthétiques*
American Edition

"Lia Schorr has been a superb source of beauty advice for the readers of *Health Magazine* and I personally follow her sound rules for healthy skin care."

—Adelaide Farah
Senior Editor
Health Magazine

"Lia Schorr's wholistic approach to skin care is one I have always admired, recommended, and used myself."

—Barri Lynn
Fashion Director
In Fashion Magazine

Lia Schorr's Seasonal Skin Care

by Lia Schorr
with Shari Miller Sims

Prentice Hall Press
New York London Toronto Sydney Tokyo

Prentice Hall Press
Gulf+Western Building
One Gulf+Western Plaza
New York, New York 10023

PRENTICE HALL PRESS and
colophon are registered trademarks of
Simon & Schuster Inc.

Library of Congress-Cataloging-in-
Publication Data

Schorr, Lia.
  [Seasonal skin care]
  Lia Schorr's seasonal skin care / by
Lia Schorr with Shari Miller
Sims. — 1st ed.
    p.   cm.
  Includes index.
  ISBN 0-13-535139-1
  1. Skin—Care and hygiene. 2. Hair—
Care and hygiene. 3. Women—
Health and hygiene. 4. Beauty,
Personal. I. Sims, Shari Miller.
II. Title.
RL87.S345 1988
646.7'26—dc19   88-310
                                        CIP

Designed by Gates Studio

Photographs by Carol Weinberg
Illustrations by Isabelle Dervaux

Manufactured in the United States of
America

10 9 8 7 6 5 4 3 2 1

First Edition

*To every woman who takes
pride in herself, in being a
woman.*

*And to my daughter, Segaal,
who continues to bring magic,
joy, and pleasure into my life
. . . and to my father, whose
presence and inspiration to
life I miss so much.*

Acknowledgments

There are many special people whose enthusiasm and encouragement helped to make this book possible. First of all, I thank Bette Schwartzberg of Prentice Hall Press, who accepted my proposal and gave this book its start, and PJ Dempsey, also of Prentice Hall Press, who took over and nurtured the project into a reality. I also thank Shari Miller Sims, who devoted her time, her talent, and her friendship to this book.

Additionally, I want to thank all those who worked to make the book beautiful, including Carol Weinberg, who skillfully photographed the interior, Kathleen Gates, whose creativity and great talent produced an exquisite design, Art Kane the magnificent cover photographer, as well as Joey Mills, my makeup artist and Sean Chin Sue, who expertly styled my hair for the cover shot.

I would also like to express my appreciation to everyone who stood behind me during the past seven years since I opened my own business—friends, family, clients, and employees, and especially members of the press, who helped me to bring needed information on skin care to a much wider audience.

Last but not least, I would like to thank my brother, Moti Peleg, for his generous personal and professional support—and willingness to be there when I need him.

—LIA SCHORR

Contents

Introduction

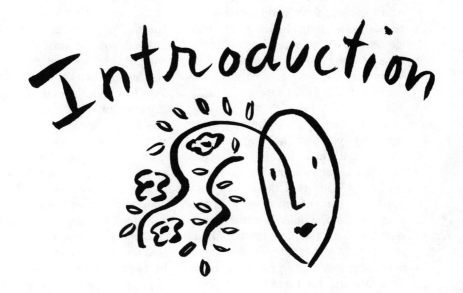

In the past few years, there has been an explosion of interest in self-care—in taking care of our bodies (inside and out) and our skin. There has also been, as those who peruse the best-seller lists or the shelves of their local bookstore are well aware, a huge increase in the numbers of books offering advice on every subject from climbing the corporate ladder to perfecting your muscle tone to—not surprisingly—taking care of your appearance and skin. Why then, you may ask, do you need another book of skin care and beauty advice?

My answer, quite simply, is that the book you are holding in your hands right now is very different from any other skin care book. In the first place, this is a book based on nineteen years of experience in the skin care field, a book in which I present the facts that are known about skin care in the modern era without any fluffery or false promises. *What also sets this book apart from other skin care books is the way in which it is organized—around the seasons and stages of a woman's life. I believe this is the most logical way to plan for your skin's needs, and leads to the simplest skin care system because it is the most realistic one.*

In short, this is a book for *all* women, of every age, every skin type, every skin coloring. It has valuable information for those women who have never paid much attention to the state of their skin but suddenly realize that time is taking its toll. It is also for women who have spent a great deal of time and money using many different types of skin care products but have never been fully satisfied with the results.

My goal is to take some of the mystery out of skin care: to debunk the myths, to simplify your choices, and to help you take the best possible care of your skin during every season and at every age. Although women spend more than $1 billion annually on skin cleansers, lotions, and potions that promise to affect the skin in possible and impossible ways, very few women who come to my salon are truly happy about their skin care routines. They complain that skin care has become too time-consuming, too complicated—or that the moisturizer that seemed to do wonders for their skin last month feels too heavy and greasy now. A big part of the problem is that *few women recognize that skin care needs to change with the seasons, with the years*, that the skin is our largest organ and is sensitive to variations in the outdoor and indoor environment, to moods, and to hormonal changes. All of this means that the skin products and cosmetics that work for a woman today may not be the ideal choices next month or next year—and that skin care should be continually evaluated and adjusted.

MODERN TIMES
Skin Help and Hazards

There is no question that the skin care products available today are light-years away from the heavy "cold creams" of the 1950s, and that modern technology has had a positive impact on the choices available to a woman who wants to take care of her skin today. But not all the advances have been without drawbacks: Preservatives and fragrances put into many skin care formulas are key causes of skin irritations and allergies, and we have lost touch with the pleasure and relaxation of natural, homemade skin care products. For this reason, you will find recipes in this book for easy-to-make skin care products included for every season of the year and every type of skin. Of course, not every woman wants to mix up her own skin care preparations at home—and the recipes I've included are not necessary to following the advice in this book. Consider them an option, a wellspring of ideas to dip into when you have the time, or the desire, to do a little "beauty chemistry" of your own.

Aside from the technological impact of skin care products themselves, modern living has also had another equally important effect on our skin: pollution. It's no secret that we no longer live surrounded by clean air and pure water. One of the biggest problems facing a woman's skin today is not only pollution but the effort to remove it from the skin through overzealous cleansing. Throughout this book, you will find valuable advice on choosing cleansing products geared to your skin type, the climate, and the changing seasons of the year. Bear in mind that the choice of cleansing products is one of the most crucial skin care decisions you can make.

SEASON-BY-SEASON SKIN HINTS

Following is a list of some of the topics that are included in this book to help you simplify and organize your skin care system throughout the seasons:

- Summer sun smarts
- Warm-weather skin smoothing
- Swimming, sweating, and playing outdoors: how to protect your skin

- Fall: moisturizers plus
- Fresh-start masks and facials
- Humidity and your skin—indoors and out
- Coping with dry skin
- Beating excess oiliness
- Winter protection—from cold, wind, and sun
- Spring refreshers: facing up to a new season
- Makeup dos and don'ts for every season and every skin color and type
- Hand and nail grooming simplified
- The seasons of your life: skin care at every age
- Hair removal: what works, what doesn't
- Pro facials: what to look for
- Getting your money's worth from skin care
- Body care, exercise, travel, and much, much more. . . .

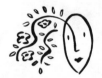

As you can see from this list, the information I've included in this book is based on real-life needs and concerns, a factor that also led me to include several question-and-answer sections in which I've addressed the most common questions presented to me by clients in my salon.

As a modern working woman, I know that the last thing most of us have enough of today is time—so I've tried to present skin care facts in a concise and easy-to-read fashion. I trust it will help you to make the most of your appearance in every season and at every stage of your life. And I hope that this book will serve as a reference source to the many generations of women concerned about keeping their skin healthy and attractive for many years to come.

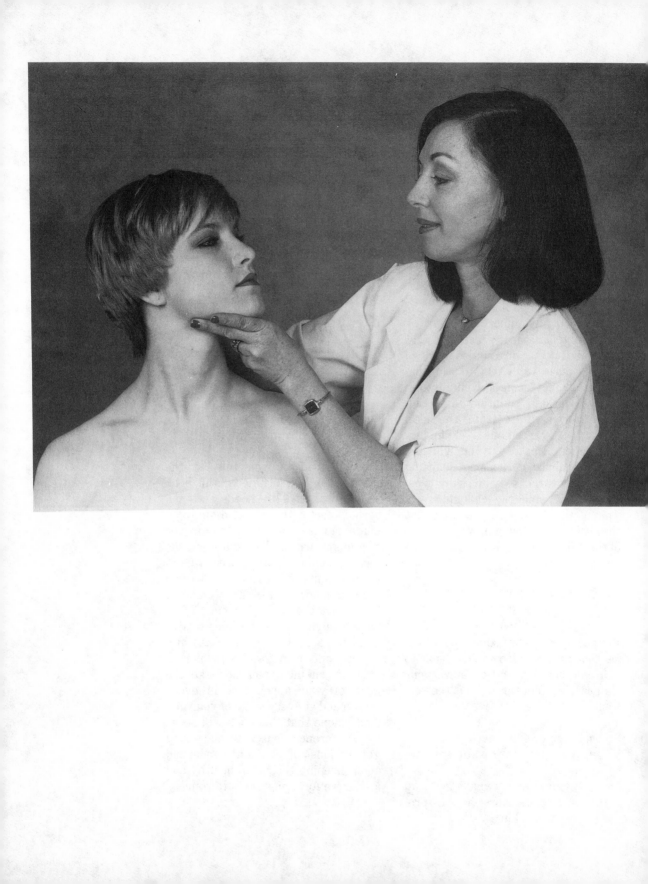

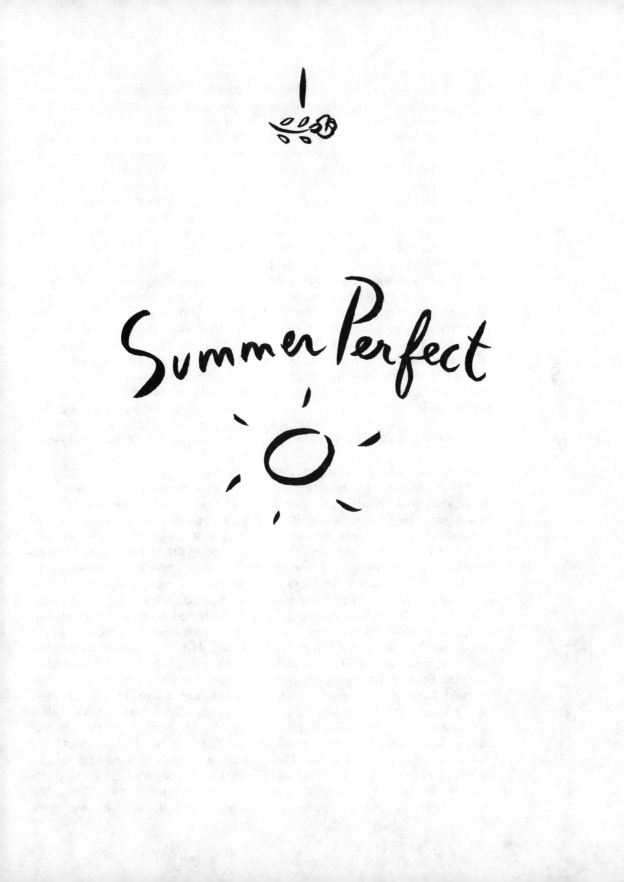

1

Summer Perfect

Summer is a season of freedom—of wearing lighter, barer clothes, of spending weekends out in the sun, of a more carefree attitude even in the most buttoned-up of corporate offices. Consider that even in workaholic offices, many companies routinely close up shop at 1:00 on Friday afternoons in summer. Everyone, it seems, knows that summer is a season of relaxation, a time to enjoy oneself. Children are home from school and every woman's fancy turns to spending time outdoors. Because of all that outdoor exposure, summer means that skin is not only on show but often takes a beating. Summer skin concerns are a combination of protecting the skin and lavishing restorative attention on moisturizing and cleansing.

SOME LIKE IT HOT

Many women who come to my salon feel that summer is the best time for their skin, that blemishes magically disappear. They need spend little time on skin care, these women insist, because summer solves all their problems. Some women who suffer from dry, flaky skin at other times of the year also feel that this is the season when their skin is at its best.

The warmth of the sun *does* have some benefits for all skin types: For dry skin, it means that the oil glands are stimulated to produce a bit more oil and thus hold moisture in the skin's upper layers. For oily skin, a bit of a tan can be the perfect blemish-drying treatment. Yet summer also takes its toll on skin in a way that may not be immediately visible but that is essential to beautiful skin in the long run: Sun exposure—the

pleasure of summer for many women—is the key cause of premature aging and wrinkling of the skin and also contributes to the more serious problem of skin cancer. Summer can be a radiant time *if* you take care to avoid oversunning, the skin's most insidious enemy. I'm not telling you to spend your summer indoors; I'm just advising you to take care to protect your skin if you want to look younger longer!

Years ago, women of the upper classes routinely avoided the sun, wearing wide-brimmed hats and carrying parasols to protect their skin from the sun's rays when they went walking outdoors in warm weather. Only farmers and laborers, who could not afford to stay undercover, sported suntans and, eventually, the weatherbeaten, old-before-their-time skin that gave testimony to years of sun exposure. In the 1920s, trend-setter Coco Chanel and a band of friends decided that they loved vacationing on the Riviera so much that a suntan was the perfect expression of their active *sportif* lives. In time, a suntan became a badge of leisure and luxury, of wealth and worldwide travel.

I myself experienced the effects of getting too much sun, having spent my teenage years living on a kibbutz in the Israeli desert and the next few years working outdoors as part of the Israeli Army. At that time, scientists and physicians had not yet alerted us to the dangers of too much sun exposure, and I thought I looked best when my olive-toned skin was taken one step deeper by sunlight. Despite the fact that we "kibbutzniks" did mix up all sorts of wonderful skin lotions and cleansers from fresh fruits and vegetables drawn from the kitchen and the garden, we knew nothing of sun protection factors or sunscreens and skin remoisturizers. After I came to the United States and lived in New York City for a while, where I could not get year-round sun exposure, I saw a change in my skin—for the better. During those years, I also learned more and more about skin care and began reading numerous articles published by dermatologists on the dangers of getting too much sun. Within a few years, when I looked at photographs of myself taken in Israel, I realized that I was beginning to look younger rather than older as time went on—namely because my skin was repairing itself as I stayed out of the sun! Medical research has now proven what I was sensing all along: While it is true that the sun works its damage on your skin over time, it is also true that once you begin to protect your skin from the sun, your body's restorative powers take over and undo some of the damage. Staying out of the sun, it turns out, may just be that fountain of youth we've all been searching for.

SUN
Cause and Effect

First suspicions of the sun's damaging effect on skin may have been caused by a single doctor observing that patients who spent their winters in warm climates somehow looked older for their ages than patients who had to toil away at jobs up North all winter long. In any case, research has now proven beyond a doubt that the sun can damage our health and appearance if taken in too heavy a dose. The good news about sun: The new sunscreens actually make it possible

for a woman to get a tan but still protect her skin from damage.

How is it possible to get a tan with a sunscreen, you ask? The answer is that the tan develops more slowly but actually lasts longer if you use the proper protection. Contrary to what many women believe, sunscreens do not block out all the rays of the sun. What they do is selectively absorb a certain percentage of the sun's damaging ultraviolet radiation before it can hit the skin. (The only way to block *all* the sun's impact is to stay in a brick house with no windows.) Although sunscreen use means that less of the sun's damage will hit your skin, some tanning rays will still do their work, turning your skin—over time—to a much-sought-after brown color. Because your tan builds up more slowly, it is less likely to peel, more likely to last. We all know too well the aftereffect of going out in the sun unprotected: a painful burn that quickly turns to peeling, flaky skin—not an attractive proposition at all.

How the Sun Works. Two types of ultraviolet rays contribute to the sun's effect on our complexions. The shorter *UVB rays* are the main cause of sunburn—and at one time were the only type of rays that sunscreens could block out. These rays are most intense at midday (from 10 A.M. to 2 P.M.), which is the reason all dermatologists and skin care experts will urge you to stay out of the sun at this time. The midday concentration of UVB rays also means that spending repeated time outdoors during these hours increases your skin's risk of long-term damage.

Until recently, it was thought that the longer *UVA rays* had little or no effect on the skin. Now it is known that, although these rays do not burn the skin, they do penetrate into the skin's lower layers, where they contribute to the breakdown of its elastic fibers. UVA rays actually cause a chemical reaction within the dermis that eventually weakens the bonds of elastin and collagen fibers—the fibers that are responsible for skin's resiliency and tautness, that is to say, its youthful appearance. Over time, exposure to UVA rays hastens the appearance of wrinkles and folds in the skin and literally ages a woman before her time.

Other reasons for the increasing concern among dermatologists and skin care experts about UVA exposure: UVA radiation, many physicians feel, is the culprit in many of the changes in the skin's immunological makeup. Exposure to UVA rays seems to set the stage in some way for the appearance of precancerous skin growths, chipping away at the skin's ability to heal itself and to fight against the development of skin cancer. Many doctors also feel that UVA radiation may be responsible for phototoxic reactions—skin rashes and blotches that appear to be brought on by exposure to the sun in combination with wearing skin lotions, fragrances, soap residues, or makeup that contain allergy-promoting ingredients. Put simply, there is a great deal of evidence to support the advice that every woman should use a "full-spectrum" sunscreen that contains ingredients meant to guard against both UVA and UVB rays.

KNOW YOUR SKIN, YOUR SUN SPOT

Selecting the proper sunscreen is a combination of your skin coloration plus your "sun spot," meaning the geographic place where you will be "taking" the sun. Obviously, the closer you are to the equator the stronger the sunscreen you will need—and the more hours you will have to stay out of the sun each day if you truly want to protect your skin.

Recent years have seen a flurry of all sorts of sunscreen formulas and have also revealed that sunscreens are even better than we had all hoped. The news now is that sunscreens can actually help your skin to repair itself and help prevent the development of sensitive skin over time. The key to their powers: Sunscreens must be chosen wisely and applied liberally and repeatedly, all over exposed skin areas whenever you are spending more than a few minutes in the sun.

To choose a sunscreen wisely, you'll need to think of tanning not as a skin beautifier but a retaliation process by the skin cells against the menace of the sun's rays. The "soldiers" in the skin's defensive action are the melanocytes—the pigment-bearing cells of the skin. Pigment can be thought of as our body's natural sunscreen, although not the world's most powerful one by any means. Pigment's screening capacity explains why it takes a good deal longer for a black woman to get a burn than it does for a white woman to succumb to sun overexposure. However, the notion that black skin is immune to sun damage is an erroneous one, as all too many of my black clients have found out when they've taken their first Caribbean vacations and come back with painful, blistery burns. Although a black woman doesn't necessarily have more melanocytes than a white woman—we all have approximately sixty thousand per square inch of skin—she does have more pigment-producing potential in each cell. Your skin color is a good indication of how "mobilized" your body's pigmentary defenses are.

In the old days, before we understood the long-term results of basking in the sun, few women thought very much about skin protection. A bottle of baby oil or "tropical coconut oil" plus a reflector was typical beach gear—and a painful burn all too often the short-term result, with wrinkled, parched skin to follow twenty or so years later. Little wonder that sunburn relievers were "hot" sellers come July Fourth!

Modern sunscreen formulas now differ greatly from the oil-laden potions of the past. We have learned now that burning is only the immediately visible aspect of getting too much sun, that the real effects go much deeper. And it is here that cosmetic and pharmaceutical chemists have come to the fore. The best way to think of sunscreens—and to get yourself to use them regularly—is as age-protectors in a bottle.

The newest sunscreens focus on speeding up the tanning process so that a woman can spend less time exposed to the sun's rays and get *more* skin color. The reason for this development: Dermatologists were finding that, because sunscreens were so effective, women were misled into thinking that they hadn't gotten any sun, so could spend more time tanning. Ironically, the advent of sun protection was backfiring: Because a woman's skin hadn't turned red, she thought she could continue sunbathing, when in fact she needed to get out of the sun to avoid the invisible damage going on below the skin surface. Now, companies have reformulated many sunscreens to include tan-promoting ingredients, enabling women to tan faster and thus spend less time in the sun to attain more of a "glow."

PLAYING BY THE NUMBERS

The key to the best sun protection is to choose the proper sun products. The system that has been worked out to help consumers in the United States make the right choices is the SPF—sun-protection factor—scale. The scale runs from 2 to 15, but some companies have introduced sun-protection products that reportedly have even higher protection—SPF 18 up through the 30s. Dermatologists and other scientists feel that these are unfounded claims in many cases, as there is no regulation by the federal government's Food and Drug Administration of sunscreen labeling at this time. In any case, the best advice is to use the highest number possible if you want the most sun protection.

Indeed, although most skin care experts advise that no woman should wear less than an SPF 8 when spending any length of time in the summer sun, the woman who is truly concerned about the look and health of her skin—and that should be you if you're reading this book—should wear an SPF 15 during this season. It is also wise to apply sunscreen ten to fifteen minutes *before* you go outdoors, to allow the ingredients to bond to the skin surface and begin to do their job. For a person who is perspiring, reapplying sunscreen every thirty minutes to an hour is not overdoing it.

The basis of sunscreen choice is your skin type, that is, your skin's ability to tan when unprotected from the sun. Below is my personal adap-

5

tation of the sun-protection scale, with an eye to the long-term smoothness and attractiveness as well as health of the skin:

Type I: Skin that always burns easily, never truly tans. Use SPF 15 at all times.

Type II: Skin that burns easily, tans minimally when unprotected. Use SPF 15 or 10.

Type III: Skin that burns moderately, tans slowly to a very light tan shade. Use SPF 10.

Type IV: Skin that burns minimally, usually tans well. Use SPF 8.

Type V: Skin that is olive-toned, can tan to a deep brown over time. Use SPF 8 or 6 (but do not use the latter at the height of sun intensity when additional protection is recommended).

Type VI: Skin that rarely burns, specifically black skin. Use SPF 6.

You will notice that I have left out SPFs 2 and 4 from my chart. This is because I do not believe that these sunscreen strengths are appropriate for summertime use. They simply do not screen out enough of the sun's rays for this time of year. Save them for spring or fall, when you can do with lighter protection, or for wearing under makeup during the summer, when the combined effectiveness of makeup plus sunscreen will be equal to SPF 6.

Another important note of caution: These SPF guidelines are intended for the strength of sun exposure at sea level in the central area of the United States. Your choice of SPF should depend on the latitude or climate. A trip to the Caribbean islands or the Mediterranean shore necessitates an increase of one or two SPFs. For example, if you have olive skin, use SPF 8 or 10 in these areas rather than SPF 6. High altitudes also call for stronger protection; the atmosphere is thinner on a mountaintop than at sea level, so there is also less natural screening out of ultraviolet radiation. Similarly, more UV radiation penetrates dry air than humid air, as the water droplets that make for humidity also deflect some of the sun's harmful rays back up into the sky, away from the earth's surface. If you plan to take a walk in the Sahara Desert, you should increase your usual SPF to 15. One client of mine who went on a vacation in the Middle East found this out the hard way: When she came back with a burn, she just couldn't understand why her usual sun-protection product hadn't done its usual job. The reason: The Egyptian sun is a good deal more intense, and a lot less forgiving, than the sun in Fort Lee, New Jersey, or the shore of Easthampton!

When SPFs were first introduced in this country, during the early 1970s, many women thought the numbers indicated how much more time they could stay in the sun while wearing a particular sunscreen versus no sunscreen at all. For example, wearing a lotion with SPF 4, many believed, would allow them to stay in the sun four times longer than usual. Nothing could be farther from the truth. An SPF 4 means that one-fourth of the sun's burning and skin-damaging rays are still getting through. In other words, it's simply poor judgment to spend hours in the sun, regardless of what type of lotion you've applied.

SUN
Separating Myth from Fact
❦

Despite the increase in knowledge among women of all ages about the effects of the sun on the skin, I find that all too many of my clients still cling to some erroneous notions about sun protection. Here are some of the most common myths, plus the reasons that these myths can be dangerous to the health and appearance of every woman's skin:

I thought I could't get a sunburn on a cloudy or hazy day. Absolutely false. Just because you can't see the sun doesn't mean the sun can't see you. On a hazy day, up to 80 percent of the sun's ultraviolet rays are still getting through. And, since the time lapse between sun exposure and visible sunburn is usually about six hours, the damage you do to your skin is not even apparent until later in the evening. The solution: Apply a sunscreen whenever you're outdoors in summer, whatever the weather.

Once I get a tan, I don't need sunscreens anymore. Wrong again. A tan may keep you from getting a sunburn, but it doesn't protect your skin from the harmful effects of sunlight that go on under the surface. Even with a tan, the lower layers of the skin are bombarded by ultraviolet radiation. Changes are occurring that, while not visible to you, are affecting the physiological structure of the skin, changes that eventually will lead to wrinkles and sagging skin twenty years later.

The only time I use sunscreens is at the beach. This is the wrong idea if you're interested in maintaining your skin's youthful look. Dermatologists caution that long-term sun damage doesn't come only from basking on the beach but also from being outdoors without protection during such everyday activities as pruning bushes, playing tennis, having a picnic, or watching a ball game. In other words, the effects of the sun are cumulative—and every minute you spend in the sun without using a sunscreen, wherever you are, is another minute you've moved toward skin that is prematurely old. Since there is no turning back the clock, the time to protect your skin is now. And it is also your responsibility, if you have children, to begin educating them about protecting their skin from damage as early in life as possible.

I thought that swimming underwater, I was protected against the sun. In fact, a full 95 percent of the sun's rays that hit the water's surface can reach your skin—even if you're snorkeling three feet under! The good news is that many of the newest sun products are formulated to be water-resistant, which means that they maintain their SPF powers for a forty-minute period of water immersion. Waterproof products will give you eighty minutes of sunscreening while swimming. These are also the sunscreen formulas to go for if you'll be exercising and working up a sweat outdoors in the summertime. More good news: Several new products have been tested for abrasion resistance, which means they won't rub off when you dry yourself with a towel after you step out of the water. Don't let these claims lull you into a false sense of skin security if you're spending the day outdoors, though; it's still wise to reapply sunscreen products every hour or two.

I thought I could buy one sun preparation for my body and my face.

This is not true. The skin on different parts of the body differs both in thickness and in sensitivity to the sun. Certain skin areas—the eyelids, lips, neck, and chest, as well as the tops of the shoulders—are especially vulnerable to sunburn. To protect the eyes and lips, look for a product that is meant specifically for use in these areas (many lip and eye protectors are packaged in lipsticklike tubes for easy portability and application). Because the neck and chest are among the first skin areas to age, even prematurely, you might want to use a sunscreen with a higher SPF rating in these areas, or put on a T-shirt if you'll be spending a long time outdoors. The tops of the shoulders, prone to burning because they are often the first spot the sun hits when beating down from above, also will benefit from extra protection.

Whenever possible, wear sunglasses that protect from ultraviolet radiation (ask an optometrist if you're unsure whether your present glasses do the job). It's also never a bad idea to wear a wide-brimmed hat or sit under an umbrella at the beach. Remember, too, to protect your skin from the drying aftereffects of sun exposure from the inside out, by drinking plenty of water (*not* beer or wine, which robs your body of water rather than replacing it).

IF YOU OVERDO IT
Sunburn Coolers

It happens to all of us—we forget to reapply sunscreen, or get caught off guard when swimming or sailing, and end up with a red, painful sunburn. If your skin is blistering, don't treat it with home care; see a dermatologist as soon as possible (or, if it's a weekend, take a trip to a hospital emergency room), as you may need to apply prescription ointments to hasten skin healing and prevent infection.

Should you buy one of the products labeled as sunburn coolers in your pharmacy? Opinion is divided among experts. Some feel that they are useful in cooling off the skin and relieving the pain. Others caution that some patients develop an allergic reaction to the main ingredient in these products—a local anesthetic—and then trade the pain of sunburn for the discomfort of a rash!

In my opinion, it's best to use natural remedies to ease sunburn pain. Here are some suggestions that I have found worked for my clients who got too much sun:

• Take a cool bath. Mix 3 teaspoons of baking soda into the bathwater to soothe the skin further. Apply tea bags soaked in cool water to the eyes (keeping eyelids closed, of course) to decrease swelling and skin sensitivity. Pat skin dry.

• Apply a head-to-toe mask of plain yogurt, which contains both cooling and skin-therapeutic ingredients. Rinse off in a cool shower; pat—don't rub—skin dry.

• Drink plenty of water to offset dehydration, a frequent result of getting too much sun. Avoid sweet drinks; your body's effort at processing all the sugar will only make your body feel warmer.

• Apply a layer of baby powder between your skin and your clothes to decrease skin friction.

• Keep your skin moisturized to inhibit peeling. *Never* try to peel away skin before it comes off of its own. It will only expose raw, sensitive skin before it's ready to face the elements. Let skin follow its own natural healing course to avoid further skin irritation.

• Don't use washcloths or loofahs until your skin has healed fully. These can exacerbate skin sensitivity and irritation.

• Make a lettuce lotion compress and apply to skin at night. Boil lettuce leaves in water; strain. Let cool in a refrigerator several hours. Dip a cotton ball into the cool liquid and press *gently* onto skin.

• Buy pure aloe vera gel or an aloe vera lotion and use as a moisturizer. The nearly complete amino acid in the juice of the aloe vera plant is believed to help stimulate skin healing and the growth of new, healthy cells.

Sun-Induced Freckles. Many women notice freckles only in summer after they are out in the sun. This is actually a reflection of the skin's effort to tan in spots where the melanin is unevenly distributed. This results in an irregular "tanning" pattern that appears to us as freckles. Many women find that by using a sunscreen with a high SPF, they can prevent freckling, but once freckles have appeared, it may take a whole season for them to fade away.

Liver Spots. Sun-induced skin discoloration is the most visible proof of how the skin alone cannot sufficiently screen out all of the sun's rays. In some cases, the skin's defensive mechanism of "pooling" pigment in particular spots on its surface leaves uneven brown patches that do not fade away with time. This most commonly occurs on the back of the hands, and we call the result *age spots* or *liver spots*. While skin bleaching creams can provide some help, the effect of these creams is not a protective one; they merely "erase"

spots temporarily, not prevent new ones from forming. Dermatologists can permanently remove brown spots from hands by freezing them away—in a technique called *cryosurgery*—or burning them away with acids similar to those used in a chemical peel. A woman with fair skin is at greatest risk of developing liver spots and should always be careful to apply sunscreen to her hands as well as to her face and body.

If You're on the Pill. Be aware that one of the side effects of being on the Pill can be a much-increased sensitivity to the sun, which can often result in edema—or swelling—of skin that has been exposed to the sun's rays. What should you do if your skin swells up after you've spent the day out in the sun? Apply ice compresses, take a cool yogurt bath, and call your physician. Chances are, he or she will recommend taking aspirin, applying cold compresses to the skin, and waiting a day or so before resorting to medication, but do check with your doctor anyway, as some reactions require medical attention. You should discuss any possible side effects from prescription medications with your doctor before venturing into the sun.

SUMMER FACTORS

The sun is not the only environmental influence on the skin in summertime. After all, most of us spend a good deal of our days indoors, too, whether at home, in the office, out shopping, or visiting friends. Each place we go, the air around us changes, and these changes, over the course of a season, influence the look, the texture, and the smoothness of our skin. Here is a look at some of summer's skin pluses and minuses:

9

Air Conditioning. A fact of life most of us appreciate in summer, air conditioners not only cool the air indoors but filter and dry it. The filtering means that skin is exposed to fewer atmospheric pollutants and stays cleaner over the course of a summer's workday than it does when you spend a great deal of time outdoors (this doesn't mean, though, that you should skimp on your cleansing routine).

The drop in humidity that occurs in an air-conditioned environment means that, although you perspire less, your skin still loses moisture through invisible evaporation. Studies show that in susceptible women, air conditioning can cause excessive skin dryness and flaking, especially if your desk or bed is located near the air-conditioning outlets. The solution: Up your water intake (drink at least eight glasses daily) and your moisturizer application. Also key: Apply moisturizer to *damp* skin—after taking a shower or bath, say—so that the oils in the cream can "lock" moisture in your skin cells. Why is this so important? It is the water content, not the oiliness, of skin that gives it its softness. Coating the skin with a film of oil via a moisturizer only helps to prevent the moisture in your skin from evaporating; it doesn't actually add moisture to the skin cells.

If you find that your skin becomes especially dry when you spend a lot of time in air-conditioned rooms at this time of year, hook up a humidifier in your home or office; you'll notice a difference in the look of your skin in the course of a day or two.

Humidity. Combined with the heat of summer air, which stimulates the skin's oil glands, humidity can prevent the skin's self-cooling mechanism from working at peak efficiency. For a woman with dry skin, the effect may not be all bad: The less moisture that escapes from her skin, the less dry and flaky her complexion will be. If your skin is sensitive, however, the salts in perspiration may act as an irritant (see next section).

If you have oily skin, humidity can promote increased skin problems, especially around the nose, where excess oiliness can give the skin a shiny appearance and blackheads can result. The solution: Rigorous—but not rough—attention to skin cleansing to remove the bacteria and pollutants that humidity can attract (see section on summer cleansing, page 12).

SWEAT AND THE SKIN
The Good and the Bad News

There are good and bad aspects to perspiration. On the one hand, sweating is the body's way of maintaining a core temperature of 98.6 degrees Fahrenheit—when body temperature rises, perspiration comes into play to cool things off. On the other hand, left to run its course, perspiration can often lead to skin blemishes and irritation.

We all know that perspiration can be annoying, even embarrassing. We always begin to perspire just when we least expect or want to, when we're nervous—about to meet someone new, for example, or to speak before a crowd. But perspiration is not a voluntary process, and while it is often a response to environmental heat, sweating can also be triggered by stress, both the emotional kind and the physical variety—for instance, the stress of combating an illness or infection or the hormonal stress of entering menopause. (If perspiration becomes a year-round or particularly serious problem, it should be checked by a physician, as it could be a symptom of a hormonal imbalance.)

While most of us think of sweating as something that goes on under our arms, sweat glands are actually spread across almost all of the body skin in varying concentrations. There are two types of sweat glands: the apocrine glands, which secrete the type of sweat associated with body odor and are concentrated in the underarm area, and the eccrine glands, which are found on the forehead, palms of the hands, and soles of the feet. Sweat glands are also found in smaller numbers on the shoulders and back.

Perspiration itself—regardless of the kind of gland it is secreted from—is odorless; odor develops from the mix of bacteria with sweat that has been secreted on the skin. The reason that sweat on the forehead rarely develops an odor is that bacteria have no chance to react with sweat in this area.

Other problems that can occur as a result of sweat that pools on the forehead are blemishes and clogged pores. When the salts that are contained in perspiration are not cleansed off the skin rapidly enough, or when sweat pools under bangs on the forehead, it is not unusual for tiny blackheads or whiteheads to appear. This is especially common among women who exercise outdoors in hot, humid weather. The solution, however, is fairly simple: If you exercise or work up a sweat in summer, always carry cotton balls doused with an astringent in a plastic bag in your purse or gym bag; that way, you

won't need to be near a sink or shower to cleanse your skin. If you forget to carry astringent-soaked cleansing pads, then at least remember to wipe your forehead with a water-soaked towel during the break between tennis sets or during a quick stop when you play other outdoor games. After you've finished exercising, cleanse your face and body thoroughly in a shower or bath and apply a scented powder or moisturizer.

Other precautions to take when the weather's warm and your activity level is high enough to work up a sweat:

• Don't wear makeup while you're exercising. Forget about vanity, forget about your appearance; all it will earn you is an irritated complexion. Makeup—whether cream or liquid formula—will trap perspiration on the skin, and the combination of the salts in perspiration and the oils and fragrance in makeup will inevitably contribute to skin breakouts. Instead, cleanse your face thoroughly before exercising. If you'll be working out outdoors, apply a sunscreen formulated for use on the face—if you're wise, you'll choose one with a high SPF. If you're heading for an indoor gym or tennis or racquetball court, leave your skin bare or apply a lightweight moisturizer; save the heavier creams for days you're not exercising. Applying a too-rich cream during exercise can cause even dry complexions to develop blemishes.

• If you have sensitive skin, be aware that blotchiness can be the skin's reaction to irritation resulting from the salts contained in perspiration. Cleanse your skin thoroughly with a gentle, creamy cleanser and avoid potentially irritating highly

11

fragranced cosmetics at this time of year.

• Be aware of the difference between an antiperspirant and a deodorant and choose the formula that's appropriate to your needs. A deodorant is merely a fragrant cover-up and will not reduce the degree of perspiration; most women find that a deodorant is a fine choice when the weather is not too warm and what's wanted is a fresh feeling rather than a perspiration-fighter. An antiperspirant, however, contains chemical compounds that work to inhibit, although by no means completely eliminate, perspiration. For best results, apply a deodorant or antiperspirant fifteen minutes before getting dressed, so the product has time to dry. Experts note that an antiperspirant can even be applied the night before, after you take a shower, and still be "active" the next morning, as long as you have not showered it off or perspired heavily overnight. In any case, remember that you'll want to avoid getting deodorant products on your clothes, as the stains can be difficult, if not impossible, to remove.

• Don't be harsh in cleansing your skin after you've perspired. One of the most frequent causes of skin irritation or sensitivity is a too-heavy hand with a cleansing sponge or cloth. Rubbing at the skin will only cause your complexion to become red and dry; instead, gently apply a cream-formula cleanser and use either a water-soaked cotton ball or repeated splashes of cool, clear water to rinse the cleanser away. Finish with several more splashes of water and pat—don't rub—your skin dry with a clean, soft towel. Also, remember to change and launder your towels and washcloths regularly, as bacteria and dirt that you have cleansed away can be unknowingly reapplied to the skin with a not-so-fresh towel.

SUMMER CLEANSING
A Skin Essential

Summer is a time for paring down, and skin care is no exception. The ideal routine focuses on cleansing away summer perspiration. Begin with a fluffy cream cleanser formulated for your skin type, rinsed off with repeated splashes of cool, clear water. If your skin tends to be a bit oily, follow with a gentle toner and a light moisturizer. If your skin is dry, a richer moisturizer is best.

Be aware that the cleanser you use in the wintertime may not be up to the job in summer, when perspiration and humidity combine to act like magnets drawing dirt to the skin. Aside from switching to a somewhat stronger cleansing formula, remember that you may need to step up your skin-cleansing routine. In winter, simply washing your face once in the morning and once at night is enough; if you are active in hot weather, you may want to cleanse your skin at midday as well. If your skin is oily, you'll want to follow each cleansing with an astringent or toner. While it might seem best to use one with a good deal of alcohol in the formula, this is not so. Alcohol can eventually overdry the skin, so choose a formula in which alcohol is not the first and most concentrated ingredient.

Deep cleansing can boost the look of your complexion at any time of year, and summer is no exception. The best way to achieve it is with a professional facial. Many women mistakenly shy away from facials in the summertime out of the false fear that the masks and cleansers used during a facial will somehow cleanse away their tans. In fact, having a facial, with its cleansing and moisturizing benefits, may actually be the best way to *extend* a tan! Likewise, many women skip facials at this time of year because they believe that a little bit of sun is all the deep-cleansing, complexion-clearing exposure their skin needs. Although this may appear to be true on the skin's surface, it is not applicable to the skin's underlayers, which is where blemishes actually begin. While the sun seems to be clearing up the skin, oily pockets are collecting under the surface, often leading to postsummer breakouts more severe than ever. You need the thorough cleansing that a professional facial can provide, cleansing that can act as a blemish-preventer all year long.

If your skin is oily, beware of pampering a tan too much. Many women with oily complexions switch to richer moisturizers once they get a tan, in an effort to prevent skin peeling. After a while, these moisturizers eventually clog the pores, leading to skin breakouts. If your complexion is prone to breakouts, stick to a nongreasy moisturizing *lotion* (not a cream) all year long. Consult a skin care professional if you are unsure of the formula to choose.

At every time of year, remember that skin cleansing does not stop at the neck. In summer, when more of the body is exposed to sun, wind, and water, it's a good idea to give body skin a thorough cleansing and deflaking by using a body sponge or loofah when you're in the bath or shower. (An alternative is one of the new exfoliating cleansers specifically formulated for body skin.) Don't neglect shoulders, back, ankles, and feet. Once you're out of the tub or shower,

lavish on a rich body moisturizer—perhaps a fragranced formula, as long as you don't have a sunburn—and some skin-smoothing, moisturizer-rich body powder. Remember to pay special "moisture attention" to the shoulders and neck.

TAKING THE HEAT
Steam, Sauna, and Jacuzzi Smarts

Summer is a time when many women enjoy the pleasures of steam rooms, saunas, and jacuzzis at home or at the health or country club. While these can be wonderfully relaxing, especially after vigorous exercise, some precautions should be followed. Cases of heat exhaustion, and even of heart attack, have occurred because of the persistent belief that if a few minutes in a hot environment is good for you, a few minutes more is even better. Here are some basic definitions and guidelines for safe relaxation.

Saunas are wood-lined rooms equipped with wooden benches in which dry, heated air is circulated. The temperature range is traditionally 160 to 210 degrees Fahrenheit. An import from the Far East, saunas are said to cleanse the body by sweating out impurities from the pores.

Steam rooms are tile-lined rooms that are steam-heated with hot, moist air kept at a temperature of approximately 180 degrees Fahrenheit. A favorite of the Finnish, who traditionally followed a session in the steam room with a dip into ice-cold sea water, steam rooms are reputed to soften and cleanse the complexion, calm the nervous system, and help the body to flush out impurities.

Jacuzzis are oversize whirlpool tubs in which the water is heated above natural body temperature. Jacuzzis are often as much a part of pro team training grounds as are locker rooms; athletes use them to massage away muscle cramps and enhance the postworkout relaxation effect.

Safety guidelines

• *Limit your stay in a heated environment to no more than five minutes per session—and even shorter if you're using a sauna, steam room, or jacuzzi for the first time.* If you want to stay longer, leave after five minutes, wait five minutes, then go back in for one or two minutes more.

Staying in a superheated environment can cause even an otherwise healthy woman to suffer from fainting spells. For this reason, it is also unwise to be in a sauna, steam room, or jacuzzi by yourself. Always have a partner who can go for help if it's needed.

• *Cleanse your skin thoroughly before taking the heat.* In a steam room, apply a light moisturizer to skin if you wish.

• *If you have very sensitive skin that is prone to broken capillaries, avoid saunas or steam rooms.* If you don't want to give up the relaxing benefits, however, bring along a bowl of ice cubes and a facecloth, and pat the skin with the cold cloth every few minutes. Limit your stay to three minutes or less.

• *If you have a sunburn, avoid heated environments—they can intensify skin trauma.* The pressure of a jacuzzi can result in increased skin sensitivity, so be sure to take it easy.

• *Wrap your hair in a towel or headband.* Keeping hair off your face avoids trapping oil on the skin. For hair nourishment, apply a cream-formula conditioner before going into

a sauna, steam room, or jacuzzi. The heat will boost the conditioning effects and help to prevent your hair from drying out.

• *After a sauna, steam room, or jacuzzi, treat yourself to a cool (but not icy-cold) shower or dip in the pool.* Afterward, apply a rich body moisturizer, and, if you wish, precede your shower with one of the following masks, to be left on for two minutes before showering.

Nourishing Yolk Mask (for the face)

Blend 1 egg yolk with 1 tablespoon wheat germ oil. Smooth over skin; wait 1 to 2 minutes; rinse off in shower.

Oil Smoother (for the body)

Combine 1 tablespoon each of wheat germ, safflower, and olive oils in a small bottle with a top. Cover and shake well, then apply to skin areas prone to dryness: shoulders, elbows, knees. Wait 1 to 2 minutes; rinse off in shower.

WATER, WATER EVERYWHERE . . .

In summer, water has both an inside and outside effect on the look of a woman's skin. The reason: The smoothness of a woman's complexion depends on its inner and outer water balance, on how much water can be drawn from the body's resources, how much can be held in the surface cells, and how much or how little you go swimming.

Water: Inner Info. When I first came to the United States and found myself surrounded by more types of junk food than I had ever imagined existed, I found it hard to resist. My willpower was virtually nonexistent, and after a few months of overindulging, both my waistline and the lack of glow in my skin told the story. So I decided to seek the advice of a nutritionist. One of the first questions she asked was how many glasses of water I drank each day. "Water!" I said. "Who drinks water? Everyone here drinks soda or coffee all day." Her advice after that first visit was to start drinking six to eight glasses of water daily. To my surprise, I not only saw an almost immediate drop in my weight—when you're drinking all that water, who has time to snack?—I also saw the return of a glow to my skin I thought I had lost forever.

It's a proven fact: To a large degree, our skin depends on our body's inner resources for its moisture—for how smooth and resilient it is. In summer, when perspiration robs our bodies of more moisture than is usually lost in the course of a day, replenishment is essential. Is water the only choice? Soda or mineral waters are also okay, so long as they have little or no sodium. Fruit juices are also fine, but stay away from tea or coffee unless they're decaffeinated, as caffeine robs the body of moisture. Avoid alcoholic beverages if you can; while piña coladas are fashionable by the seaside, they not only deplete the body of fluids but go to your head a great deal faster in the heat of the sun than they would in other environments.

Water: Swimming Smarts. Swimming is just about the ideal exercise for every woman. Suspended in the buoyancy of fresh or salt water, the muscles and joints of the body are perfectly cushioned to avoid stress or injury. But swimming can have a not-so-favorable effect on skin and hair. Here are tips on avoiding skin or hair dryness from too much of a good thing:

Always use water-resistant sunscreens when you're heading for a dip in the pool or ocean. Countless times, I have received telephone calls from clients who were almost in tears because of an extremely painful sunburn, yet claimed that they didn't even sit in the sun. When I asked what they were doing outside all day, they inevitably answered, "It was so hot; I was in the pool." The next question: Were they wearing a sunscreen tested for water-resistance? "No. I didn't think I could get a sunburn in the water." The truth is you can—and it can be a bad one. Always use a sunscreen formula labeled *water-resistant* or *waterproof*. (See the earlier section of this chapter dealing with sunscreens on page 5.)

Rinse off as soon as you get out of the ocean or pool. Chlorine and salt can be damaging and drying to skin and hair, and blondes know all too well that chlorine can give their hair a greenish tinge (ask your hair-salon staff to recommend one of the new conditioning formulas meant to prevent this). If you can't find the time for a shower, then just dip under cool water from a showerhead for a few seconds—the rinse-off effect will be pretty much the same, and certainly better than no rinsing at all.

If you swim a great deal, change your moisture routine. This means that you'll need a richer moisturizer, a more intensive conditioner for your hair, aimed at offsetting the inevitable drying effects of too much salt or chlorine.

15

GORGEOUS HAIR
Protection Counts

In warm weather, *carefree* and *easy* are the words that capture the style of a woman's hair. Summer is the time for a haircut that works, one that is easy to take care of, falls into place with a minimum of fuss. None of us wants to be a slave to curling irons or hot rollers in hot weather. Many women go for a shorter hair cut in summer for this very reason: There's no need for setting or for frequent visits to the beauty salon, often no need even to use a blow-dryer! A layered cut, today, can be designed to fall into place when wet and look smashing when your hair dries in the warm summer breezes. For those times when you want a more "finished" look, gels, mousse, or hair spray can help you achieve it.

One of the problems of summer: Just when you're depending on your hair to look great in any weather, the environment is trying to dry out and damage it. Sun exposure and swimming can weaken hair; humidity can lead to frizziness, air conditioning to dry, split ends. The solution is intensive conditioning once a month and the use of an instant conditioner after every shampoo. If you'll be spending a great deal of time sitting outdoors, try to wear a hat. And if you can't stand hats, then provide your hair with some additional protection by applying a creamy conditioner before you sit in the sun for an extended length of time. Or use one of the new hair sprays or gels that have sunscreens built into the formula. The best in-sun conditioning method is to wet your hair (by jumping in the pool, for instance, but coming out after a minute, before damage can occur, and then rinsing hair with cool water), apply a cream conditioner, then wrap your hair in a turban-tied towel. The towel will "reflect" body heat back to your head, boosting the conditioning benefits.

Avoid blow-drying or using hot rollers too often in summer, when hair can be more fragile and vulnerable to dryness because of sun exposure. When hair is wet, gently comb it. (Don't brush it—brushing wet hair can stretch it to the breaking point.) Use mousse or gels to set hair in place. When it's very hot or you're exercising, always keep hair off the face, especially the forehead, where hair can trap sweat and skin oils and lead to unwanted blemishes.

"HELP! MY HAIR TURNED GREEN!"

If you're a blonde, chances are you've been the one to scream out in horror as, after a day in the pool, you glanced in the mirror and saw that your hair had taken on a greenish cast. The cause is the algicides added to swimming pools to retard the growth of algae, which often contain copper compounds that interact with the chlorine in the water to form a greenish deposit on the hair. Wearing a bathing cap that fits well enough to keep out most of the water is one way to prevent the problem, but there is very little that you can do at home once it occurs. The best bet is to go to a beauty salon and ask the colorist for help. *Don't* try to color your hair in an effort to cover the green yourself—it will only become more of a mess. (Hair that has been bleached blond is also at risk of turning green in a swimming pool, so do wear a bathing cap when you swim, and consult your professional colorist should anything go amiss.)

COPING WITH COLOR
OR PERM

Hair color and perming processes have greatly improved since the days when coloring your hair meant that your hair would take on a dry, straw-like texture. Today, questions about the safety and "kindness" of hair color treatments and perming are answered reassuringly by physicians, who note that many of the ingredients once thought possibly harmful to a woman's health have been replaced by substances proven to be safe. Today, having beautiful hair means having hair that is in good condition—shiny, full, and attractive in every way. At top salons, conditioners are blended into customized hair color formulas; at home, hair color kits sold by major manufacturers now include conditioners that are either blended into the hair-coloring mixture or applied immediately afterward. Yet, despite all the good news, colored or permed hair *still* requires additional protection from sunlight, which acts as a natural bleach, damaging hair made more vulnerable by chemical processes.

If you've spent several days in the sun without wearing a hat or coating your hair with a conditioner, chances are you've ended up with hair that looked dried out and brassy. What causes brassiness? Peroxide, which is not only an ingredient in just about all hair-coloring products (and a major ingredient in those that work to lighten hair) but is also contained in perm neutralizers—the solutions applied to hair to stop the perming process and lock in a certain degree of curl or wave. Even if the peroxide has been thoroughly rinsed out of your hair before you go into the sun, once your hair has been treated with peroxide in perm or color, it no longer has the same degree of structural integrity and will be more vulnerable to the effects of the environment—heat, ultraviolet light, and wind.

What to do to "cure" brassiness? One option is to visit the professional who did your color or perm, for fast repair. But if there's no time for that—if you need help immediately—the best solution is to buy a *nonperoxide* toner (available wherever hair color is sold), apply it to the hair for five minutes after shampooing, then rinse it out with cool, clear water and apply a deep-conditioning pack, which should be left on the hair for fifteen minutes. The toner will reduce the brassiness, and the conditioner will improve the texture and feel of hair, as well as its smoothness and shine.

Don't make the mistake of attempting to cover up brassiness by using a darker-toned coloring product. While it may work initially, even darker hair color formulas often contain some peroxide, usually in the toner, as a way to brighten hair even when it's dyed darker, which means your hair will become more damaged and brassy within a week or two after its use.

SUMMER MAKEUP
Less Is More

In summertime, we all wear light, airy clothing in pale tones or icy pastels. Makeup should have the same light touch, the same breezy appeal at this time of year. The biggest mistake women make in summer is to wear the same makeup they wear in winter; the cardinal rule of summer makeup is that less is indeed more—less makeup allows a woman to feel more comfortable, lets the skin "breathe," and helps a woman to

17

show off the beauty of well-cared-for, sun-touched skin.

For these reasons, it's a good idea to make a special effort to look for light, sheer makeup formulations at this time of year. Look for water-based foundation, lightweight loose powder, and sheer lip colors. Colors that let the texture of your natural skin come through are best. If you do have a bit of a tan, choose makeup that shows it up, doesn't hide your skin. Think in terms of powder eye shadows and blusher; creams not only feel less comfortable on the skin in warm weather but also tend to "pool" in skin creases and take on a "cracked" look by midafternoon. In terms of color, this is the season when peach tones, soft corals, lilac, soft pink, sun-dappled rose, and sea-foam green are especially flattering. Stay away from aquamarine and light blue—they're old-fashioned and will make even a young woman look older and out of style. In choosing specific shades, it's always smart to take a look at several fashion magazines before you go to the stores, to see what's in fashion this season. Then, at the store, try to sample colors whenever possible, as it's sometimes hard to tell which will be most flattering against your skin when you look at a color in its package. Take advantage of free makeup lessons whenever possible (in many department stores, the cost of a makeup lesson is credited toward the purchase of cosmetics). Ask questions of professionals about specific methods of application that will be most flattering to the shape of your face and your skin texture and tone.

While the notion of matching your makeup to your clothes is somewhat outdated, it is true that a woman should always be aware of the ways in which cosmetics can *complement* fashion, play up the colors in a floral patterned dress, say, or playing down the harshness of neon tones. In general, today's basic makeup rule is "anything goes," but try to work with your natural skin tone in choosing foundation and blusher, eyeshadow and lipstick colors. If your skin tends to take on a yellowish cast, you'll want to stay away from cosmetic shades in the yellow family—such as peach or apricot—as they can emphasize a sallow complexion. Similarly, if you have a classic "Irish" sort of ruddiness in your complexion, you might want to stay away from colors that are too reddish, or pink or purple shades, which can emphasize the redness in a less than flattering manner.

DAYTIME BEAUTY

In summer, as in every season, there are two basic makeup looks: the natural look and the more dramatic look. Chances are, you know instinctually which you prefer; both looks can be stylish in every season, and some women vary their choice depending on what they have planned for each day. At this time of year, both looks should begin with a sheer, liquid-formula foundation in a color that is as close to your natural skin shade as possible. (When shopping for foundation, don't make the common mistake of matching it to the skin of your hand, which can be several shades different from the skin of your face. Instead, test a new foundation shade on your neck, which is closest in color to your face.) For the most natural finish—and longer-lasting makeup in humid weather—apply foundation using a makeup sponge, preferably one with a triangular shape that can be used to blend out the foundation at the hairline and edges of the chin. If you use powder—and women who truly want their makeup to last throughout the day really should—you'll want to choose a translucent loose powder at this time of year, applied with an oversize makeup brush (a natural-bristle brush is best), then dusted off with the same brush to remove any excess powder.

In summer, it's a good idea to choose matte powder eye shadows and blusher and matte cream lipsticks. If your lashes are pale, you might consider getting a lash tint—basically a matter of dying your lashes a deeper color using a nontoxic natural dye without coal tar. This process should always be done professionally at a skin care salon by someone who is aware not only of the proper technique but of the necessary precautions to protect the delicate skin around the eyes. Because two lash tints will last all summer, you'll never have to worry about mascara that runs in hot weather. If you choose not to have a lash tint, you'll want to use waterproof mascara at this time of year, when the humidity and heat can "melt" regular mascara formulas.

If you like *soft, natural makeup*, then chances are you'll want to choose a monochromatic makeup palette, basically a matter of selecting blusher, lip, and eye shadow shades all within the same color range—all shades of peach, pink, or soft brown-beige. Start with a sheer foundation as above, followed with a brush of translucent powder, if you wish. Then, using either a soft peach, pink, or beige powder eye shadow and a sponge-tipped eye shadow applicator, apply shadow over the entire eyelid, from the base of the lashes up to the

brow bone. The color should be most concentrated near the base of the lashes, palest on the brow bone. Then, apply a lavish coat of mascara to top and (if you wish) bottom lashes, waiting until the first coat is dry before applying a second one. Using a soft, natural-bristle blush brush, apply a soft coral, pink, or brown-beige powder blusher to the tops of cheekbones only, using a round line of application. Blend out the blusher with a tissue or soft powder puff so there is no obvious line of demarcation (what you want is a soft tinge of blusher on your cheeks, not a noticeable stripe or round circle of cheek color, one of the most common makeup mistakes). Finish with a matte lipstick in soft pink, coral, or golden beige, blotted with a tissue. If you want a bit of translucent shine, touch your finger to a pot of clear lip gloss, then to the center of your lips.

For those women who prefer a more *dramatic look*, choose a more contrasting makeup palette, with cosmetics applied with more definition. Begin, as above, with a translucent liquid foundation matched to your skin color, and "set" it with translucent loose powder applied with an oversize makeup brush. Then use a sponge-tipped applicator to smooth on soft pink, peach, or beige powder eye shadow from the base of the lashes up to the brow bone, concentrating the deepest color near the base of the lashes, with the softest color near the eyebrows. Use a deeper, complementary powder shadow (sea green with the pink, chocolate brown with the beige, apricot with the pale peach) to accent the eyes; with a sponge-tipped applicator, dot on shadow at the outer corners of the eyes, then blend down to a smudge of color with the fingertips.

Choose an eye pencil in the same shade as the deeper-toned shadow and use it to line the eyes close to the base of the lashes—for the most smudged line, dot on color close to the lashes, then use a cotton swab to blend the dots into a soft-edged line. If you want to accentuate the eyes more, do the same under the lower lashes. Finish eyes with mascara on upper and lower lashes, then use a round natural-bristle brush to apply powder blusher in a soft pink, rose, peach, or brown-beige shade matched to your skin tone. Keep blusher high on the cheekbones and use a tissue or sponge to blend it out until there's no obvious line of demarcation (no matter how dramatic you want the overall effect of your makeup to be, what you don't want is a clownlike appearance to your blusher). Use a matte lip color in a rich pink, soft red, or coral shade (don't use mauve or purple shades in summer; they take on an unattractive cast in natural sunlight). If you want a more defined mouth, use a lip pencil in the same shade as your lipstick to line lips first, then fill in with lipstick and blot with a tissue.

EVENING ATTRACTIONS

Summer evenings are usually less formal than at other times of year: Evening clothes are barer, somewhat more casual, and there's a greater freedom, too, to evening makeup. The main difference between day and evening cosmetics in summertime is that, at night, you can add a bit of shine to catch the sparkle of summer moonlight.

The guidelines for application of makeup at night are generally the same as during the day, except at night you can choose a more opalescent eye shadow, a foundation with built-in sheen, or a metallic lip color. The one rule: As in daytime, less is more. You'll want to go for a touch of shine, not an allover metallic effect. If you want a bit more, then keep the same makeup application as in the day, and finish with a light brushing of a glistening translucent powder over the edges of the forehead, cheekbones, nose, and chin. There are now a wide range of glittery powders that can also be brushed onto shoulders, the hollow of the neck, even the décolletage at night. Let your destination be your guide: If you'll be inside in brightly lit surroundings, then a slight tinge of shine is all you'll want. If you'll be outside in sparse candlelight, a bit more shine can be alluring. One new and very appealing option: Scented glistening gels, which add sparkle and fragrance to bare skin in summertime, can be a fast way to go from day to evening when there's no time to take off the old makeup and put on the new.

SPECIAL OCCASION
Makeup for Summer Brides

Every woman wants to look her best on her wedding day. Her makeup should be as perfect as her hair and wedding gown, but it is equally important for a bride to feel comfortable with her look. If you are not used to wearing very much makeup, this is not the time to experiment with an overly made-up style. If you want to have your makeup done professionally for your wedding day, as many brides do, it is essential that you try out the makeup artist beforehand. You'll want to be sure that the makeup artist's style is one that you like, and that the look you get on your big day is the one you had in mind. If, on the other hand, you are one of those brides who chooses to play it safe and do her own makeup, the following suggestions will help you achieve the perfect look.

If you usually wear little or no makeup, then consider using soft pastel colors applied in a very natural-looking manner. Think of soft pink or cream or sherbet yellow powder eye shadow smudged subtly from the edge of the lashes to the brow bone on each eyelid, with an eye pencil in the same color as the shadow used to deepen the color slightly just above the lashes. A soft powder blusher in pale rosy pink or soft coral plus a matte lip color (stay away from too-deep shades, as they'll appear even darker in photographs) will finish the look.

If you like the look of a bit more color in your makeup, add a touch of a contrasting powder shadow in a slightly deeper shade—sea foam green, apricot, golden yellow—at the outer corners of the eyes, and a deeper-toned pencil in the same color family to line upper and lower lids softly. Don't use black eye liner, though; it will photograph terribly and make you look as if you have two black eyes.

Which brings us to a very important point when considering makeup for the bride and her attendants: Be aware that the camera can play tricks with your makeup, and work to take advantage of the camera rather than be shocked by it. What to do: Avoid a shiny face; the light will bounce back at the camera, making your features look blurry and your skin greasy. To avoid this, use matte—not iridescent or frosted—shadows and blushers as well as lipsticks, and finish your makeup with a generous brushing of matte translucent pow-

der (a bonus of this powdering is that your makeup will last longer). Stay away from lip gloss; use creamy matte lipstick, applied over a base of matte concealer for longer-lasting color. Don't make the mistake of applying too much makeup out of fear that you'll look washed out in the photographs. A professional photographer will have already adjusted the lighting and camera settings for regular "street" makeup, so any theatrical techniques will end up giving your face an overly harsh, overly made-up look in the wedding album. Do pay attention to blending out all color—especially blusher, so you don't end up looking like a clown with stripes of makeup on your face. The general rule: If in doubt about your makeup, remember that less is more.

FAKING A TAN

The secret behind many a perfect, year-round tan is a tube of bronzing gel, the best way to supplement the skin-saving use of sunscreens. With a bronzer, you can get a little sun and come back with a lot of tan—or so everyone else will think. I predict that ten years from now, when more women and men heed the warnings of skin specialists about how bad the sun can be to skin's health and appearance, more than half of all Americans will get their tans from a tube.

"But a bronzer looks so dark and my skin is naturally fair. How can it possibly look natural?" I hear you ask. A bronzer only looks dark in the tube; it is formulated to become translucent on the skin and to let the natural tonality of a woman's complexion come through. Unlike a foundation, which is a cream or a liquid, a bronzer is a gel, formulated to be sheer, to adjust, so to speak, to your skin texture and tone. Because bronzers are nongreasy in formula, they can be used by women with every type of skin—dry, combination, or oily.

Bronzers come in stick or tube form. I prefer the tubes because they contain lighter gel formulas, whereas the sticks have more of the heaviness of foundation. Start with a very small amount squeezed into the palm of the hand and rub it onto your face using your fingertips. Be sure to blend quickly and well; blending is absolutely essential for achieving a natural look with a bronzer, and if you blend fast, you won't have any streaks. Be especially sure to blend out the color at the hairline and along the edges of the chin. Also be sure to apply bronzers before getting dressed, to avoid staining the collar of your clothes.

Don't overuse a bronzer; it will give your skin a dark brown "wooden" appearance. Let a bronzer substitute for both foundation and blusher to achieve the most natural look. Like any other makeup, bronzer should be washed off the skin before exercising to help prevent skin breakouts.

SUMMER VACATIONS
Beauty Basics

If you're lucky enough to take some time off during the summer to head for a vacation spot, chances are you'd like to travel light. No matter how concerned you may be about your appearance, the idea of dragging along all of your beauty supplies is never an appealing one. Nor is the notion of spending hours of your precious vacation time fussing with skin care or makeup. Here is a list of the minimum "beauty basics" you can bring

on vacation. You'll never need anything else (See page 203 for a longer list).

- Toothbrush and toothpaste
- Liquid rinse-off skin cleanser
- Sunscreen formulas in various SPFs
- Foundation (water-based is best)
- Darker translucent powder (to substitute for foundation if you get a tan, or help to "fake" a tan while you use lighter foundation)
- Waterproof mascara
- Eye crayon (a "fat" eye pencil can double as liner and shadow)
- Neutral lip color

A frequent traveler's trick to simplify packing: Keep a separate travel-only makeup kit packed at all times containing the above essentials. All you'll need to add is a miniflacon of your favorite fragrance of the season and you're ready to go. After each trip, make sure to clean out the kit and update the color, say, of your foundation or eye pencil. Where's the blusher, you may ask? Every woman carries one in her purse every day, so that's the one to use when you travel! In any case, if you're heading to a sunny spot, once you spend a day outdoors, you won't even need to use a blusher!

QUESTIONS OF
THE SEASON

Q: I notice that my skin often looks shiny by the end of the workday in summer. How can I apply my makeup so that this doesn't happen?

A: In warm weather, many women do not need to wear a

moisturizer plus a foundation. You may want to switch instead to a tinted moisturizer—basically one that contains a lighter concentration of the coloring ingredients used in foundation. In addition, it's a good idea, if your skin goes shiny by late-day, to apply a light dusting of translucent powder with an oversize makeup brush in the morning, after you've applied the rest of your makeup, and to touch up the powder later in the day.

Q: There seem to be more and more "instant" or "pretanning" tanning products on the market. Can these products truly give you a tan without the harmful effects of the sun? Are they safe?

A: Basically, all "instant" or "pretanning" products contain one of several ingredients that act as a skin dye. All of the lotions on the market that claim to give you a tan without the sun or accelerate the tan you get within minutes in the sun contain either derivatives or chemical synthetics of the ingredients that give carrots their orange coloration. While this makes the products, in one sense, "natural," it also means that your skin will look orangy yellow, rather than brown, after using these products.

Instant tanning products are all relatively safe. While a few women may find that they are allergic to instant tanning formulas, for most women the main drawback in using these lotions is that the resulting "tan" is very unnatural-looking. It's a good idea to test the product by first applying it to the inside skin of the arm; that way, you can both check for an allergic reaction and see the coloration the product will give your skin.

Once you use these products, you can not usually wash away the results. The natural ingredients seem to penetrate the skin cells so thoroughly that soap can't remove them. One positive note: Because the ingredients do their instant-tanning work on the very outermost layers of the skin, the body's natural exfoliating process will rinse away the dead skin cells, and the orangy color, within a week or so.

Q: How can I prevent or lessen the skin dryness that follows a day spent outdoors in the summer?

A: The perfect summertime refresher is a tall, cold glass of water. It's the only way to replenish skin moisture from the inside out, which is where it really counts.

After spending time in the sun, take a lukewarm—not hot—shower and pat your skin with a towel until it's not quite dry. Then lavish on a rich moisturizing lotion, preferably one containing aloe vera or cocoa butter, two excellent skin soothers.

For additional natural moisturizing benefits, before you take a shower, rinse your face with cool water, pat dry, and apply a plain yogurt skin "mask." Wait fifteen minutes, then rinse off in the shower.

If your body skin becomes flaky or ashen (a frequent problem for black women at this time of year), mix up a gentle skin scrub by combining a sprinkle of sea salt with a half-cup or so of baby oil or olive oil. Use a soft washcloth to apply to body skin; rinse off with warm water. Follow your shower with a rich, fragrance-free body cream.

Q: I love using eye and lip pencils to apply makeup after a day at the shore, but find that they often melt in my totebag. What can I do to keep them from melting?

A: Try storing your makeup pencils in the refrigerator the night before you go to the seashore. That way, they're less likely to melt by the end of the day, so long as you take care to store them inside a locker or another place out of direct sunlight during the day. In summer, it's also a good idea to put all pencils into the fridge for a few minutes before sharpening them, so they don't crumble because of the heat.

Nail polish can also become a victim of excessive heat at this time of year, so try to store yours in the fridge as well. Not only will the polish be less likely to clump up, it will also go on smoother and last longer.

Q: Can swimming help my skin's circulation and improve my complexion?

A: While swimming rates among the top overall exercises—because it helps to condition the heart and lungs, as well as the body muscles, with very little risk of injury—it is unproven that exercise can have a direct impact on the look of the skin. Many experts do believe, however, that the boost in body circulation that follows exercise similarly benefits the circulation to the skin. One thing that is certainly true is that swimming in salt or chlorinated water can be detrimental to your complexion if you do not rinse yourself off soon after you come out of the water. Always rinse off with clear water after coming out of the sea or pool, and always wear a waterproof sunscreen when you go for a swim. This way, you'll prevent swimming from damaging your skin's appearance and may even find, like many exercisers, that getting into shape has visible results in the smoothness and glow of your skin.

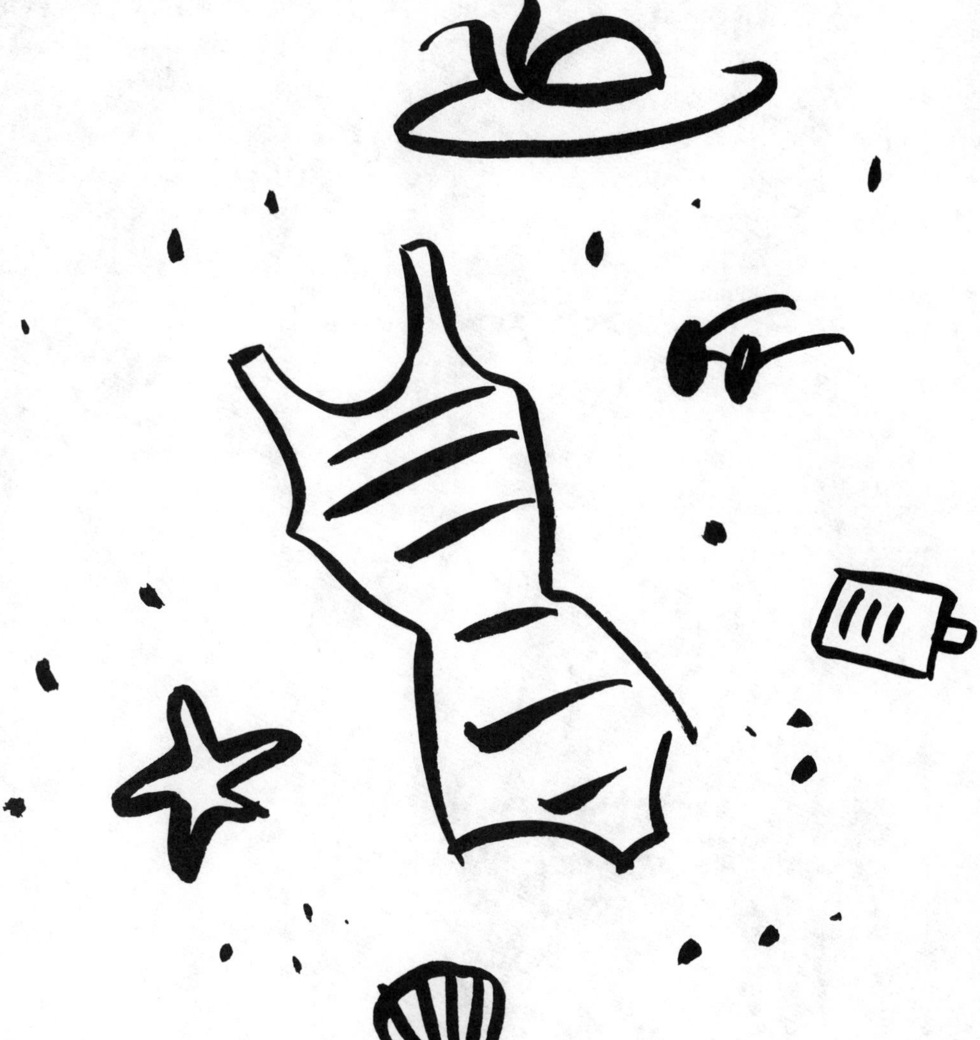

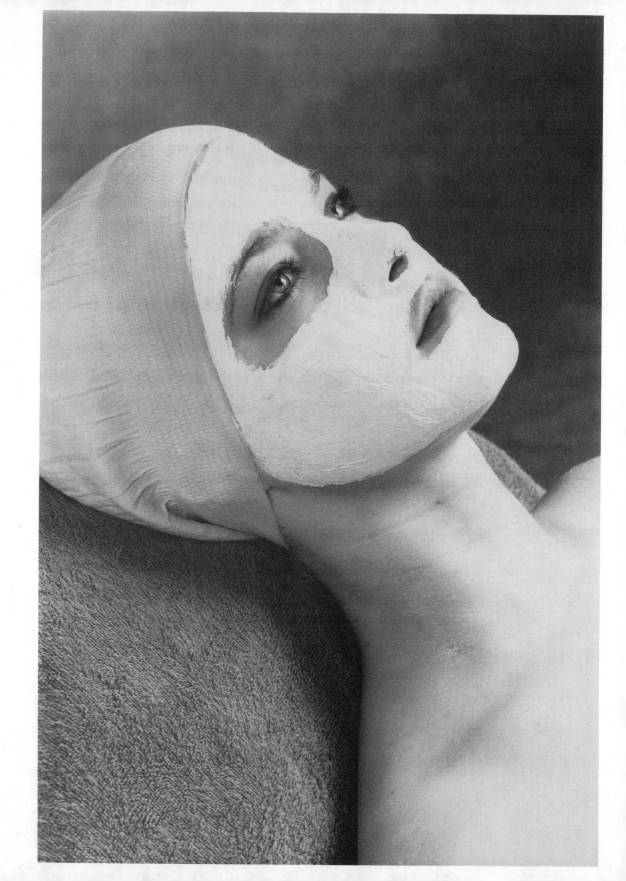

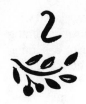

2

Foolproof Fall

Fall is a season associated with the return to routine: coming home from a trip; assuming regular work hours; going back to school—in short, putting summer's easy pace and recreations behind us. Even a woman's skin tends to "normalize" in fall, when the air is neither too hot nor too cold, and a woman's complexion not overly oily or dry.

But to *ensure* that this will happen, you will need a skin regimen that helps your complexion recover from the abuses of summer. The after-effect of tanning, swimming, and general outdoor exposure is often peeling, flaking skin. Add to that the fact that the air becomes a bit cooler and drier in the fall, and you can see the importance of "clearing away the old and getting on with the new" in skin care.

THE MOISTURE FACTOR

As the air cools down at this time of year, it also loses some of its ability to hold onto moisture, which means that more moisture is robbed from the skin's surface. The first step in maximizing skin moisture is increasing your body's water intake by drinking at least six to eight glasses of pure, clear water a day. The next, and equally important, step is to use a creamy, milky skin cleanser rather than a harsh, drying soap. Look for a cleanser that contains ingredients such as aloe, lanolin, and urea, as these all help skin cells hold onto precious moisture.

Use your cleanser gently, applying it with a damp cotton ball (*not* a tissue, as paper products can cause microinjuries to the skin surface). Rinse your skin thoroughly with lukewarm, then cool, water. And

gently *pat* your face dry with a towel. Don't follow your cleansing with a harsh, alcohol-based astringent or toner at this time of year; even oily complexions may find these too drying. Instead, look for an alcohol-free formula, or make one yourself (see the recipe for Lettuce Essence Lotion later in this chapter, on page 31.)

If you feel that your skin needs extra help, consider getting a professional facial, which is the gentlest way to slough off dead skin cells and prepare your skin for the season ahead. A professional treatment is an essential if you are left with blackheads or skin irritations after summer is over; you do not want to run the risk of self-treating these skin problems at home. If you don't have the time for a professional treatment, another good choice is to give yourself a minifacial at home. This can include gentle, careful skin steaming but it should *never* include squeezing or picking at the skin, which not only can exacerbate skin breakouts but can leave you with permanent, unattractive scars.

Steaming has been touted as a "pore-opener," but this is really not the case. Facial pores do not open and close like a closet door; pores do not have muscles, so are incapable of this kind of movement. What steaming actually does is *soften* the skin through superhydrating it; softer skin often lets go of impurities and becomes slightly plumper. Both of these factors combine to help lessen the appearance of enlarged pores.

Follow these directions for safe at-home steaming:

1. Cleanse your face with a gentle, creamy cleanser. Apply a moisturizer to protect delicate capillaries during steaming.

2. Fill a large china or porcelain bowl with boiling water (don't use a metal bowl, as this will keep the water at too hot a temperature). Add lemon juice or a soothing herb such as chamomile if you wish.

3. Drape a large, clean towel over your head and shoulders in a tentlike fashion, directly over the bowl.

4. Keep your face at least 10 inches away from the water. Getting too close to hot water during home (or even not-so-professional salon) facials is a major cause of broken capillaries, skin irritation, and acne.

5. Steam for no more than 5 minutes, taking minibreaks from the steaming every one-and-a-half to two minutes.

6. Blot your face dry with a fresh towel, then apply a rich moisturizer.

7. If your skin is sensitive, limit your steaming session to two minutes, no longer. You can safely steam your face once or twice a week, depending on your skin's sensitivity. Oversteaming is *not* better than no steaming at all; in fact, it is likely to be irritating for every skin type.

SMOOTH SKIN
A Clean Sweep

If you are like many women, you may have gotten a bit too much sun this summer, with the result being that your skin feels tough and looks a bit older than it does at other times of year. One of the newest ways to smooth and deflake skin is with a light peeling treatment. Light peels come in gel, powder, or cream form for use at home or in a skin care salon. I find that the formulas that are massaged off the skin—the cream or the powder—are preferable to the gel, which is lifted off of the skin in a film. These treatments help to re-move the dead outer layer of skin gently but thoroughly. They should not be used at home if your skin is sensitive; a skin care expert should evaluate your skin first to see if it can take these treatments.

A light peeling treatment is not to be confused with a skin scrub or exfoliating cleanser containing rough particles. These scrubs are really intended for skin that tends to break out; they are meant for cleaning out pores and discouraging blackheads and whiteheads. While a peeling treatment sounds harsher, it is actually a gentler treatment than a scrub, as it removes dead cells only from the skin's outermost surface. A scrub, on the other hand, mechanically exfoliates the skin and goes beneath the outermost skin layer. A scrub can be used on the oily T-zone of the face if you have acne-prone skin but should not be used on active blemishes, as it can spread infection.

For those women with uneven pigmentation, extreme sun damage, or a dull, old-looking complexion, there is also the option of a cosmetic deep peeling treatment done in a skin care salon. These treatments are not as harsh as dermabrasion, but may be risky if done by untrained persons. Before having a deep peeling treatment in a salon, ask the salon personnel how often they do such treatments and, if you wish, whether you can speak to other clients who have had the treatments done in the past. These treatments take six days to perform, during which time the skin will look a bit red, as if you were sunburned. The skin cannot be cleansed during this time, nor can makeup be applied. At the end of six days, the top four layers of skin will have been removed, leaving skin looking rejuvenated and renewed; the benefits often last up to a year, during which time your skin will look smoother and younger than usual, and makeup will go on more easily as well. The mixture used in my salon is a vegetable-based formula with natural enzymes and a small amount of light chemical additives; I do not believe in totally chemical-based formulas, as these can be more dangerous.

Done properly, deep peeling treatments should *not* be painful. A light burning sensation during the five minutes after the solution is applied is all that should be felt. I recommend against such treatments if you are currently taking tetracycline or other antibiotics, or if you are being treated for a systemic disease (unless you get clearance from your physician first). For the first week after the treatment, the skin should be moisturized often and cleansed *very* gently. After a week, you can resume your usual skin care regimen.

BODY BUFFING
Head-to-Toe Skin Caring

The switch from warm to cool weather requires more than a switch in facial skin care; it also means it's time for pampering body skin as well. Many women find that their skin undergoes seasonal switches, with dryness on the elbows becoming more severe at this time of year, or breakouts occurring on the chest or the back. I always emphasize to my clients that fall is a transitional season, and that the care you give your skin now will be beneficial in how your skin will look later in the wintertime.

Cooler weather makes the idea of taking a warm bath more inviting. To stimulate skin circulation, use a loofah or body sponge to cleanse your body, and follow a bath with an application of a rich body lotion. Consider adding a fragranced oil to the bath, and following up with a skin-stimulating rubdown with an oversize Turkish towel. Treat your feet to a ten-minute soak in warm water plus Epsom salts, then smooth away rough skin with a pumice stone. To keep elbows smooth, use a sea sponge plus a creamy cleanser to wash away flaky skin in the bath or shower. And bear in mind what one female client told me: She always judges a woman's true age by the look of the skin of her elbows, as it is never hidden under makeup and thus is the most "honest" skin of all.

A FRESH START
Fall's Skin Bounty

One of the most frequent questions asked by clients of my skin care salon is how to have the smooth complexion of a fashion model. While a clear complexion is partially, of course, due to heredity, it is also true that most models take very good care of their skin; they come to skin care salons regularly for professional treatments and practice good skin hygiene and care at home. And they take the time to treat themselves to a facial mask on the average of once a week.

While you may not have the time or the desire to spend as much time on your complexion as a fashion model, treating your skin to a mask made from the seasonal fruits will not only help your skin's appearance but can also give you a quiet few minutes to yourself, to relax and replenish your energy. For this reason, you'll probably want to choose a quiet time, at the end of the day or on a Friday afternoon, to turn off the lights and relax while the mask penetrates and refreshes your skin. Place a thick cucumber slice or a chamomile tea bag soaked in cool water over each closed eyelid to relieve tiredness and puffiness at the same time.

The following masks work for all skin types:

Banana Royale
Mash 1 whole banana in a small bowl. Add 1 tablespoon of honey and a few drops of orange juice. Mix to form a paste. Apply to clean skin. Relax for 15 minutes, then rinse with cotton dipped in lukewarm water. (The banana calms and nourishes the skin, while the honey and orange juice remove flaky surface cells.) Pat skin dry with a soft Turkish towel; apply a moisturizer all over face.

All-American Apple Mask
Core and cube 1 apple. In a blender, purée with 2 tablespoons honey and ½ ounce chopped sage (or ⅙ ounce dried sage). Apply and leave on face for 15 minutes. Rinse off with warm water. Pat skin dry with a soft towel; finish with a gentle moisturizer.

Masque Magenta
Mince 1 medium-size raw beet in a food processor or by hand. Mix with a few drops of heavy cream. Blend into a smooth paste. Apply to clean skin; relax for 15 to 20 minutes. Rinse off with cool, clear water. Pat skin dry with a damp towel. Apply a rich moisturizing lotion.

After you have used a masque, always cleanse skin very gently, using a gentle cream cleanser and a non-alcohol toner such as my Lettuce Essence Lotion.

Lettuce Essence Lotion
Find the darkest-leaf lettuce you can and boil leaves in enough water to cover. Let cool and strain. If you wish, add the juice of one cucumber. Refrigerate for several hours before using, preferably overnight. Apply to skin gently with a clean cotton ball.

BEAUTIFUL HAIR
Fall Is the Season . . .

Even women who recognize that it is important to adjust their skin care routines to the differences of the season often forget that the same principle applies to hair care. At this time of year, our hair often tells the tale of a summer of swimming and sunning: It is not uncommon for the ends to be dry and strawlike, the color to be a bit bleached out, and the result to be hair that is hard to manage. Taking a few extra minutes to care for your hair on a daily basis can make the difference.

The first concern should be having a good haircut. Since there is only so much that can be done to repair split ends, I usually recommend that clients who spend a good deal of time outdoors in summer schedule a haircut for the end of the season, to snip away dry ends and give hair a good shaping. No conditioner or hair treatment can replace the benefits of the right cut. Seek out a hairdresser who understands your needs—such things as your hair's texture, your life-style, your exercise schedule, and your image. You'll want a cut that makes it easy for you to style your hair at home but still allows for versatility— the ability to change the look of your hair, for example, at night.

For many women, the aftereffect of sunning and swimming in summertime is a *dry scalp*, which is often mistaken for dandruff but is actually a natural shedding of dry, dead skin cells. This is the perfect time of year to have a professional scalp treatment that will smooth away dead surface cells from the scalp and restore much-needed moisture to scalp and hair. All of the scalp treatments in my salon include a gentle steaming treatment that encourages the nourishing, moisturizing ingredients of a specially selected scalp mask to penetrate and replenish missing moisture. Also a help in avoiding a flaky scalp: Brush hair thoroughly with a clean brush before shampooing (your brush should be "shampooed" each time your hair is) and massage the scalp gently with fingertips (*not* nails) during shampooing. If you want to use a conditioner, choose a "light" (that is, nongreasy) formula and concentrate it on hair ends and underlayers to avoid a greasy buildup on the surface of the hair shafts.

If your scalp is very dry, I recommend a *hot oil treatment* at home as a supplement. This involves heating olive or vegetable oil in a glass bowl, then parting your hair in several spots and using a cotton ball to apply a small amount of oil directly onto the scalp. If possible, it is ideal to give yourself a hot oil treatment at the start of an evening at home; then you can give the oil several hours to penetrate into the skin of the scalp. After a few hours, the oil should be shampooed out of your hair and off the scalp; several rinses will ensure that all of the oil is removed. What will be left behind is smooth, soft skin and lightly conditioned hair.

Many women mistakenly believe that the arrival of cold weather signals a need to double up on hair conditioning treatments in an effort to avoid static electricity. *Overconditioning of hair* is not the answer; too often, it simply leaves hair looking oily and stringy. Instead, use a light conditioner and try to build in habits that can prevent static electricity. If possible, avoid blow-drying your hair and let it air-dry instead. Spray a small amount of hair spray onto your brush before using it; the spray will "calm" the static hairs and leave your hair looking smooth. Avoid curling irons at this time of year; they can add to the static electricity problem.

Be aware that your habits can be reflected in the look and thickness (or lack of it) of your hair. Crash dieting, illness, drug abuse, irregular menstruation can all contribute to hair loss or at least to a lack of fullness. Smoking, lack of exercise, and an unbalanced diet can also rob your hair of healthy-looking shine. Be aware that no shampoo or conditioner can do as much for your hair's appearance as can healthful habits, but it is also true that even the most "clean-living" woman can still have fine, thin hair. I myself have always had very fine, limp hair, but in the past five years, after regularly having intensive scalp treatments that include a placenta-based scalp mask, I have noticed a real difference in my hair's appearance. Obviously, these treatments have not really been able to grow more hair (nothing available without a prescription now can do this despite all sorts of advertising claims) but my hair does *look* thicker, which is what counts after all. One point of reference, however: We all normally shed between fifty and one hundred hairs a day. The number naturally ebbs and flows with the seasons, but it just so happens that fall is peak shedding time for all of us, so don't be upset if you notice that the hairs that come out in your brush are a bit more plentiful at this time of year. If your hair is healthy, it will grow back as the winter approaches.

Whatever your hair's texture or condition, be aware that too much teasing, coloring, perming, or setting can wreak havoc on its shine. Try to do as little as possible to your hair and the reward will be evident in its lush look. Beware of the tendency for shampoos and conditioners to build up on the hair shaft and leave your hair looking oily; rinse repeatedly after every shampoo and conditioning and make the last rinse a cool to cold one. Cool water will increase your hair's shine and gently stimulate the scalp.

SMART EYE BEAUTY

The dry air and winds that arrive with fall can be irritating to a woman's eyes. To keep your eyes feeling comfortable and looking clear, try to rub them as little as possible and to apply eye makeup with care. Never sleep with mascara on; it can wear off during the night and irritate delicate eye tissue. Before going to sleep, always remove all eye makeup with a specially formulated conditioning eye makeup remover. Don't use soap, as it can dry out lashes and irritate eyes. If your lashes tend to be dry and sparse, look for oil-based eye makeup removers that are meant to lubricate and "nourish" lashes. If you opt for a liquid eye makeup remover, apply it with a wet cotton pad, not a tissue, which can be too rough for the delicate skin around the eyes.

Should you use waterproof mascara? While it certainly offers a neater look than regular mascara, I feel that the ease gained is at the cost of lash fullness, as waterproof formulas can be extremely drying to the individual lash hairs. Also, despite claims to the contrary, most waterproof mascaras are difficult to remove, which means that you may end up rubbing—and irritating—your eyes in an effort to get all of your makeup off at night. Much better to risk slight smudging of your mascara during the day, which can easily—and quickly—be removed with the help of a dampened cotton swab.

One of the most frequent problems women complain to me about is difficulty in applying mascara, or in keeping it looking fresh all day. I frequently advise them to consider a professional eyelash tint, which involves applying a nonirritating, vegetable-based color to the hairs of the lashes to give them what looks like a perennial coat of mascara. This is a treatment that is especially practical for women with light blond or pale brown hair, as their lashes often appear invisible unless they are made up with repeated coats of mascara. Unless you have a history of allergies or have had a recent eye infection, the gentle vegetable dyes used in an eyelash tint should not cause any problems, but do be sure that the salon that offers this service has had experience with eyelash tinting; the tint should be applied with care taken not to get the dye into the eyes. In general, the results will be a bit exaggerated during the first evening after the tint, when you should avoid washing your eyes. Once the dye has "settled," though, you can rinse your eyes with cool water and the dye will take on a surprisingly natural look—so natural, in fact, that many men who would sooner be caught dead than wear makeup come to my salon regularly for eyelash dying. As a general guideline, eyelash tinting can be repeated once a month, although many women find that the results actually last much longer, and that they can come in for a repeat tinting once each season.

FALL MAKEUP
The Colors of the Season

In summer, a bit of sun on your face is all you need to have a healthy look, but in the fall, when natural color has disappeared from your complexion, makeup becomes a much more important beauty tool. This is not to say that what you'll want to do is pull out every cosmetic from your vanity table and use them all. In fact, I believe that the biggest mistake most women make is to use *too much* makeup. Learning to use makeup subtly, for enhancement of your own best features, is key to looking good at every time of year (see chapter 15).

What many women want in the fall is a look that will complement the heathery, natural tones of fashion. At this time of year, tweedy clothes become popular again, with shades of khaki, brown, rust, and navy often top choices. For a woman with a pale complexion, what is needed is a soft makeup palette; for a black woman, fall's clothing choices can inspire a touch of pink or soft coral in makeup. The idea for every woman is to learn to use the shades that are most flattering to her own skin tone and apply them in the subtlest manner possible.

Foundation. A key makeup choice is foundation. Rather than trying to extend the look of a tan by going for a shade darker than your complexion, I believe it looks much more natural to match foundation precisely to your skin tone or, if you want a dif-

ference, to go one shade *lighter* than your natural skin tone. Opt for the sheerest, most lightweight formula that provides the coverage you need. Depending on the texture and smoothness of your skin, you may need a bit more coverage, but you'll want to avoid products that produce a heavy, masklike look. Many women like to apply foundation with their fingertips; that's fine, so long as you use a sponge or cotton ball afterward to blend the foundation completely. Pay special attention to the jawline and cheekbone areas, where lines or streaks of foundation may be left. To give your makeup a professional-looking finish, apply translucent, colorless powder over foundation, brushing the excess away with a clean, oversize brush.

Blusher. The key to finding a blusher that flatters your skin tone is to choose a shade that complements your foundation. Avoid very bright orange or very bright red; most women find them hard to wear—and hard to apply without looking harsh. *Don't* apply blusher in a round circle on the cheeks; this is probably the most common and unattractive makeup mistake I see. You'll want to heighten your own natural color, not paint on a pair of rosy red cheeks! For the same reason, I think most women achieve better results by using powder blushers than they do with cream formulas, which require more care and blending to look natural. Unless you have exceedingly dry, crepe-papery skin, powder blusher will probably look best. Use a large blusher brush to stroke on color along the edge of your cheekbones; then, using either a clean brush or the soft edge of a sponge, blend out the color until it is barely there. If you feel the result is too subtle, then reapply a touch of blusher in the same manner again; reapplying rather than over-applying color is key to a natural-looking result.

Eye makeup. In eye makeup, fall basics include shades of gray, brown, and taupe eye shadow, with eye crayons in the same shades used for lining the eyes. You'll want to achieve a soft, dusted look, not a heavy, outlined eye. For highlighting the upper lids, think in terms of complementary shades of soft pink, palest yellow, gold-toned khaki. Many cosmetic companies offer these complementary shades together in a single eye makeup palette. For the softest application, use a sponge-tipped applicator to apply color, further blending the color with the pads of your fingers. Use the darkest shade on the lids of the eyes, the paler highlighting shades up near the brow bone. Again, take care not to overapply color for the most flattering result. To line the eye, use the softest eye pencils you can find to ease application and blending—and to avoid tugging at the skin around the eyes, which can speed the appearance of wrinkles in this delicate area. Dot on single accents of color near the lashes, then smudge together and soften with a small brush or a cotton swab. Don't rim the eye in a straight line of color; this inevitably looks unflattering and old-fashioned.

Lip color. Fall lip colors range from red to pink to coral, with just about every color in between. The neatest looking lip color begins with lining the lips in a shade that is matched or slightly darker than the lipstick shade you will be using. The lipstick is used to fill in the color; then lips are blotted with a tissue as a final step. The newest looking lip colors, while bright or vivid, also have a touch of translucency, revealing the natural texture of a woman's skin underneath. What you don't want is a solid, opaque coloring that hides the shape or texture of your lips. For a sheerer daytime lip, consider lining *and* filling in lips using a lip pencil; the result is a softer, more muted coloration that many women prefer during the day. For the longest-lasting lip color, sandwich a layer of translucent powder between two layers of lip color—or use a sheer layer of foundation as the underpinning for lipstick.

QUESTIONS OF THE SEASON

Q: Is it a good idea to have a facial at the beginning of the fall—or will it erase any remaining color I have after my summer tan fades?

A: Fall is the ideal time to have a facial—which, contrary to belief, can actually help your skin to hold onto any remaining color from the sun by smoothing out the skin surface and slowing down the peeling process.

If you suffered from a sunburn, however, you'll want to be sure that the facialist is aware of this and that she treats your skin very gently. Sunburned skin can remain sensitive for quite a few weeks, so you don't want any harsh manipulation of the skin afterward.

The deep cleansing and gentle steaming and moisturizing that are part of the best professional facials are just what most women's skin needs at this time of year—and a good facial can help to prepare your skin for winter, increasing its moisture-holding ability and natural defenses against the cold, dry air.

Q: Is a bath or shower a better idea during the fall?

A: Whether a woman takes a bath or shower is not as important as how she treats her skin before, during, and afterward. While it is true that a bath robs the skin of more moisture than does a quick shower, adding moisturizing bath oils to the bathwater can compensate for this in most cases. And a too-hot shower can be as undesirable as a too-hot bath.

What is key if you have dry skin is to apply body oil before you get into a bath, and to moisturize the skin while it is still damp as soon as you step out of the bath. The same applies to postshower skin care: Moisturizer should be applied after your skin has been patted—not rubbed—dry and is still slightly damp. By locking in skin moisture right after a bath or shower, you can turn these cleansing treatments into moisture-boosters for skin, which is very important to your skin's appearance at this time of year.

Q: My house is very dry and I am afraid that this is increasing my dry skin problem. Is there anything I can do?

A: A very well-known dermatologist was once quoted as saying that "the same environment that is ideal for a houseplant is ideal for the skin." His point was that skin smoothness benefits from a "greenhouse" environment, being surrounded by warm, moist air. During the colder months of fall and winter, it is true, the air tends to hold much less moisture than during summer and spring—a factor exacerbated by steam heating of houses, which dries out the air further. To compensate, I suggest using a humidifier to boost the moisture content of the air and help your skin to hold onto moisture within the cells.

Other helps: "double-dosing" your skin with moisturizer after a shower or bath by applying a moisturizing cream or lotion, then waiting five minutes, and reapplying it. Never skip moisturizer under your makeup, and pay special attention to areas prone to dryness, such as the tops of the cheekbones. Use a loofah gently during a shower or bath to remove dead skin cells from the surface of your body; then follow up with a rich body cream, layered onto problem areas such as knees, elbows, and feet. In general, you'll want to make more moisture available to your skin and use lotions and creams to help lock in the moisture for as long as possible.

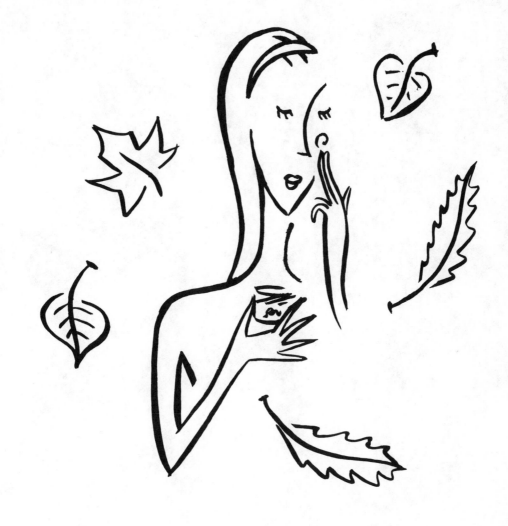

3

Winter
Wonderful

When the thermometer drops, the winds pick up, and the Christmas decorations transform every American town into a winter wonderland, few of our thoughts turn automatically to skin care. Yet winter is the season that puts our skin to the harshest test. During no other time of year is the body faced with as many challenges—moving instantly from 20-degree weather outdoors to 70-degree temperatures indoors, from cold, rainy streets to dry, overheated rooms. What makes these challenges so especially harsh on a woman's complexion is the fact that the skin acts as our body's first defense against the weather, taking the brunt of winter's icy air.

It is not uncommon for women to come to my salon at this time of year complaining of skin that is so chapped that it is painful to the touch, or of a complexion that is so flaky and dry that it looks twenty years older than in any other season. Even women with oily complexions begin to notice dry patches on their cheeks or chins at this driest time of year. For women with sensitive skin, winter is an especially cruel season, a time when nothing seems to take the sting out of their skin.

MOISTURE
Not a Drop to Spare

A lesson that we all learned in grade school is vital to an understanding of your skin's condition at this time of year. Remember, cold air cannot hold as much moisture as hot air. Moreover, heating systems are just as likely to rob moisture from your skin to increase the humidity in the indoor air.

The result: winter skin—dry, drier, driest.

What should you do about these inevitable winter conditions? Fight back with your own moisture-builders. Start by installing a humidifier wherever the air is dry—in your office, your bedroom, your den. Lower the thermostat a notch. Drink plenty of fluids to "nourish" skin's moisture needs from the inside. Finally—and most important—literally double up on moisturizer at this time of year by applying a single layer to damp skin, waiting five minutes, and applying a second protective layer. Whatever your skin type, this is also the season to switch to a richer formulation, one made to safeguard your skin's precious water quotient.

Be gentler in your cleansing routine. Shy away from harsh high-alcohol toners, for example, and opt for an alcohol-free formula. Because the cold and wind strip the skin of its natural fluids and emollients, it is essential that you not use any harsh products.

In wintertime, it is also essential never to go outdoors immediately after washing your face—the shock to the skin will only lead to chapping. Instead, wait a half-hour to allow your skin to "normalize" before heading out into the cold. *Never* go outdoors right after using an exfoliating cleanser in the wintertime; you will only end up with a red, irritated complexion.

It is very important, whatever your skin type, that you keep your skin lubricated during the wintertime. *Lubricated* does not mean saturated with water—that is impossible to do from the surface and, as I have already noted, only leads to chapping. Instead you need to "trap" the

40

water inside the skin cells in order to keep them soft and smooth. Accomplish this with moisturizer plus a moisture-retaining foundation formula. If you are in your twenties or older, winter is also a season in which wearing a protective eye cream becomes more essential than ever to prevent premature wrinkling and dryness of the skin around the eyes (it's a good idea, all year long, to choose an eye cream that contains a sunscreen if you'll be spending any time outdoors).

What to do if your skin feels very tight and dry? Indulge it with a supermoisturizing treatment, using a cream that is rich in petrolatum (*don't* use one that contains lanolin—it may cause an allergic reaction). And avoid washing with soap, as it can accelerate skin's moisture loss, causing soap dehydration and contributing to a tight, dry feeling. Instead, use a rich creamy cleanser specifically formulated with emollients that soothe dry skin. Apply the cleanser with a cotton ball, not your fingers, for germ-free cleansing.

If you are a skier, remember that the combination of drier air at high altitudes and the wind created by the rapid descent down a ski slope can exacerbate winter-dry skin. *Always* wear a sunscreen when you go skiing—snow is highly reflective of the sun's damaging rays, and wind and fog can boost the sunburn quotient by bouncing around harmful ultraviolet rays in the atmosphere. I advise all my clients to wear an SPF 15 sunscreen in a moisturizing base; even if your skin tends to be oily, it's best to save the alcohol-based formulas for summertime. As in summer, it's wisest to reapply sunscreen every half-hour to an hour, especially when

you are very active. To protect the delicate skin around the eyes from the harmful rays of the sun, apply an eye cream containing sunscreen and wear dark ski goggles that absorb ultraviolet light (ask your optometrist if you're unsure whether the goggles you have do this). If you want to stick with your usual sunglasses, avoid those with metal frames; they will transmit cold back to the skin, not only making you feel colder but robbing the skin of more moisture as well. Bear in mind that your neck, chin, and ears are especially vulnerable to chapping and sunburn, and apply rich moisture-based sunscreens to these areas, boosting protection with a scarf and hat.

You'll notice that throughout this chapter I've advised using a richer moisturizer at this time of year. What if you dislike the feel of thicker creams on your skin? Then look for one of the new lighter-weight formulations, many of which contain natural herbal-based moisture extracts and can be just as effective as their heavier counterparts. Don't make the mistake, however, of failing to use a moisturizer in winter. You will only end up regretting it when your skin loses its smooth texture and ends up flaky and noticeably dry. One possibility, though, is to use a lighter moisturizing formula during the day under your makeup and to use a richer cream at night, applying it to clean, still-damp skin before going to bed. While most women think of night cream as something that is greasy to the touch and unattractive to look at, the newer formulas are actually absorbed into the skin instantly and are virtually invisible within minutes after application. The newest night creams feel lighter because they contain nonoily moisture-holding ingredients—a factor that makes them wonderful for use, too, during cold-weather sports, when the skin needs extra protection.

BROKEN CAPILLARIES
Winter Danger Zone

One of the hazards of winter for women with sensitive complexions is the tendency to develop broken capillaries, which show up as tiny, spidery, red lines on delicate skin and are most likely to occur around the nose and cheek areas. While we use the word *broken* to describe these blood vessels that suddenly appear on the surface, in reality they are damaged rather than broken. Most women who tend to develop broken capillaries have fair, thin skin—skin that is easily sunburned or chapped by the wind. The problem is especially common in red- or blond-haired women of northern European descent (particularly the British and Scandinavians).

The precise cause of broken capillaries is not known, but some factors that seem to be associated with their appearance are overexposure to heat or cold, overconsumption of alcoholic beverages, highly spiced foods, or liquids that are excessively hot or cold, and exposure to a highly concentrated heat source. An extreme sun- or windburn may also increase the likelihood of developing broken capillaries—and a tendency to get these tiny red "spider veins" is a very good reason to protect your skin from the environment at all times.

Sensitivity to cosmetics can exacerbate broken capillaries and add to skin irritation, so it is wise to stick to a gentle range of moisturizers, cleansers, and makeup products if your skin has this tendency. Avoid mixing different brands or types of products together and try to stay away from highly fragranced formulations, since fragrance is a common skin irritant.

Is it possible to increase the resiliency of thin skin and avoid the tendency to develop this problem? Not really; genetics is the most important reason that broken capillaries occur, and, since we can't go back in time and change our inherited skin types, there is little to be done on this score. If you are a thin-skinned person, what is essential is that you take special care to protect your skin from any extreme: Use a moisturizer as a barrier between the skin and makeup; always wear a sunscreen in winter as well as summer when you'll be spending time outdoors; and avoid cleansing the skin with very hot or very cold water, relying instead on a gentle cream cleanser and a lukewarm water rinse. It's a good idea, too, to avoid the use of washcloths or harsh abrasive sponges or scrubs and always to alert skin care salon personnel before they begin giving you a facial that you have this problem. Avoid saunas, steam rooms, and tanning salons—all of these environments are certain to be highly irritating, even disastrous, for sensitive skin prone to broken capillaries.

Is there anything that can be done to rid the skin of broken capillaries? A cool mask of calamine powder plus plain yogurt is a good skin-calming treatment, as is a gentle gelée mask. A well-applied foundation can help enormously in camouflaging broken capillaries, and attention to skin protection can keep the problem from becoming worse. In severe cases, a dermatologist can use a variety of methods to eliminate broken capillaries (a simple injection is one possibility; freezing, or cryotherapy, another) but these should always be discussed carefully with a physician with the understanding that in many cases this is a skin problem that will eventually recur.

I advise clients who complain to me about broken capillaries to use the following gentle skin mask, not only in winter but all year round, once a week.

Skin-Saver Mask
Mix a small amount of chamomile powder (available in a health food store or at many skin care salons) with buttermilk into a rich paste. Apply to areas of skin that are especially sensitive (around the nose and on cheeks, but not too close to eyes); wait 15 minutes; rinse off with warm water and soft, pressed cotton.

SHOWERS AND BATHS
Getting the Winter Beauty Benefits

In wintertime, many women who are prone to dry skin find it necessary to compromise between their desire to take a daily shower or bath and the reality of their skin's excessive moisture loss. The problem: Every time you take a bath or shower, the skin's moisture balance becomes upset, with the frequent consequence that you leave a watery environment with much less moisture in your skin. While I am not advocating staying dirty in winter, I do think that a woman with dry skin needs to adjust her bath and shower routine at this time of year, switching to different types of skin-cleansing and restorative products.

What to do: Avoid long soaks in the tub at this time of year, as they in-

evitably dry the skin. To keep from robbing the skin of essential body oils, never make the bathwater hotter than 104 degrees Fahrenheit and lace the bathwater with body oil (avoid bubble bath mixtures as they are usually drying to the skin). Instead, take quick baths and use a rich body mousse to cleanse the skin rather than a drying antiperspirant soap. In the shower, try to use lukewarm rather than super-hot water and a shower mousse rather than harsh deodorant or detergent soaps. As soon as you come out of the shower or bath, wrap yourself in a big, absorbent Turkish towel and pat the skin dry. Then, immediately apply a rich body cream from the tops of your shoulders to the tips of your toes. The cream will lock in the moisture and keep your skin from drying out quickly.

In cold weather, never take a bath or shower immediately before going outdoors—the shock to the skin will be too great. Instead, allow at least thirty minutes between showering or bathing and stepping outside (this is wise advice, too, if you don't blow-dry your hair but let it air-dry, but more on that later).

While it may seem that I am maligning the pleasures of the bath, I really am not. I am well aware that through the ages, the bath has been a ritualistic beauty treatment. Marie Antoinette added buttermilk, wild thyme, and marjoram to her bath water, whereas Madame Tallien, an acclaimed beauty in the Napoleonic age, credited her flawless skin to regular bathing in a tub filled with pounds and pounds of squashed berries. What I am trying to emphasize now is the idea of wise bathing—bathing that will help protect winter skin from excessive dryness rather than

43

exacerbate the problem. Further advice: When possible, bathe in soft rather than hard water, as the calcium carbonate that makes water hard can also combine with soap to form a drying film on the skin. If the water in your community is hard, add a water-softening bath oil to soften the bath and improve the effect on your skin. *Don't* add salt to the bath water; while some people believe this has a water-softening effect, the impact on your skin will be disastrously drying, not to mention potentially very irritating. If you want to boost the skin-softening impact of a bath, hang a cheesecloth bag containing bran, oatmeal, or almond meal under the faucet as you run the bathwater.

Some soothing old-fashioned "recipes" for relaxing or skin-smoothing baths:

• Add a teaspoon of dry mustard to the bath; the result is a muscle-soothing elixir.

• If you want the relaxing effect of a fragrant bath, add a few drops of essential oil (jasmine, rose, orange, or neroli) to the bathwater.

• To soothe irritated or wind-chapped skin, add 1 or 2 cups of dry-fat milk to the bath, supplemented, if you wish, with a fragrant essential oil.

• For superdry skin, slather your body with a very high grade olive oil before stepping into the warm bath. After a five-minute soak, use a loofah briskly to rub down your skin and rub away dry, flaky cells (don't do this if your skin is very sensitive, though).

• If your feet are tired, add a handful of fresh or dry herbs (lavender, sage, thyme, marjoram—alone or combined) inside a cheesecloth pouch to a warm bath. Pour a bowl of boiling water into the tub. Wait a few minutes, until the water cools to 100 degrees Fahrenheit, then sit on the side of the tub and soak your feet for about ten minutes before going into the bath to cleanse your body.

• A skin-stimulating bath mixture to have on hand in the fridge: Heat a few cups of cider vinegar to just boiling. Add a handful of fresh or dried herbs (chamomile, sage, and rosemary are particularly appropriate); and let simmer for five minutes. Remove the pot from the stove and cover; let sit overnight. Strain the liquid and refrigerate. Add about ¼ cup to a warm bath.

• Use your bath time for special restorative skin treatments. Apply a facial mask before you get in the tub and wait ten to fifteen minutes before gently rinsing it off. Or simply mash up a fresh papaya and apply it to your face. The enzymes in the fruit will slough off dead skin cells and leave your face rosy and shining. An alternative, if a papaya is out of season where you live: Mash one quarter of a raw potato with sour cream to make a rich paste. Apply to skin; wait ten minutes; rinse off with clear water.

• Use the tub to do "bathercises," increasing circulation not only to your heart but to your skin. First, draw a warm bath and mix in Epsom salts for natural muscle-relaxing. To release tension from the shoulder blades, kneel on a rubber mat in the tub and sit on your heels. Clasp your hands behind your back with palms touching, lift your elbows, and extend your arms behind you. Hold for thirty seconds. Unclasp and arch back slightly. Sit cross-legged in the middle of the tub. Shrug both your shoulders up to your ears as you inhale. Then drop your shoulders and exhale. To loosen the ligaments that hold the spine together and stretch the muscles of the rib cage, kneel on a rubber mat in the tub and sit on your heels. Hold onto both sides of the tub for support (this is *essential*). Twist your torso to the right. Keep your chin up and hold this position for five seconds. Repeat to other side. Breathing rhythmically and deeply, repeat this movement twisting five times to each side.

WINTER AND A WOMAN'S HAIR
Protection is Key

To keep your hair shiny and healthy-looking at this time of year, you'll have to adjust your shampooing and conditioning routine. For most women, that means using a somewhat richer, or less drying, shampoo—say, one with a built-in conditioner or formulated for delicate rather than oily hair. Even if your hair tends to be oily, chances are it will be a little less so in winter than in summer. Also essential in this season is regular conditioning. The reasons: Cold air and winter winds zap moisture from hair, increasing static electricity, causing split ends, and often drying out the scalp as well as the skin. What to do:

• Use an instant conditioner after every shampooing, even if your shampoo formula has a built-in conditioner (rinse the conditioner off immediately after applying in the latter case).

• Use a deep-conditioning treatment pack on your hair once every seven to fourteen days.

• Never let your hair blow freely in the wind unless it is cut very short. If long hair flies around in the wind, it will get snarled and possibly break when you try to comb it. Either tie

your hair back in a ponytail or a braid or tuck it inside a hat for protection. If a hat tends to flatten your hair, try an underhat "set", using tube-shaped rollers to hold your hair in a chignon.

• Apply a hot-oil treatment weekly to restore moisture to hair. After a thorough rinsing, vigorously massage the scalp to stimulate circulation.

• Don't overbrush your hair in winter; this increases the likelihood of static electricity.

• Invest in a humidifier to decrease static electricity; or place a pan of water in each room.

• If you find that a wool hat causes flyaway hair, switch to an acrylic or knitted cotton one instead.

• Don't leave home with wet hair; the cold air will cause split ends and, if the temperature is below freezing, can even break hair strands.

• To control flyaways, simply rub a minute amount of styling gel into the palms of your hands, then gently stroke it into hair. Use a hard rubber comb or a brush with natural bristles rather than metal combs or plastic-bristled brushes at this time of year. Another flyaway controlling tip: Spray a small amount of hair spray directly onto the bristles of your brush before giving hair a final brushing; this is especially wise right after blow-drying in winter. (Blow-drying is a proven static-electricity producer, so allow your hair to air-dry indoors at this time of year as often as possible.)

• To get the most out of your shampoo, give your hair a real soaking before you shampoo. Use warm water to "open" the outer cuticle of the hair shafts, thus allowing the hair to absorb the beneficial ingredients of the shampoo.

• If you find that your hair is very

difficult to comb through after shampooing, use a cream rinse—a thin, light-textured liquid intended to make hair softer, shinier and easier to comb when you step out of the bath or shower. By detangling the cuticle, cream rinses flatten out the hair shaft and allow it to reflect a greater amount of light than it would otherwise.

WINTER DRY SCALP
Why It May Not Be Dandruff . . .

Many women develop what they think is dandruff in the wintertime, but is actually a dry, dehydrated scalp. Just as cold air, wind, and lack of moisture in overheated rooms can dry out your complexion, they can have the same effect on the skin of the scalp. What results is a grayish white flaking that is not dandruff but has the same unattractive consequences.

What should you do if your scalp often becomes dry in wintertime? Eat foods rich in vitamins A and D, which seem to have a preventive effect. Use a light conditioner immediately after shampooing, and take a few seconds to rub the conditioner into your scalp before rinsing. Avoid using heavy gels or pomades on hair, which can cause sweating in an overheated room (perspiration is one cause of the buildup of dry skin cells on the scalp). To close the pores of the scalp and prevent postshampoo flaking, finish every shampooing with a cool, rather than hot, rinse.

Don't apply greasy creams to the scalp in an effort to moisturize the skin; they will only lead to greasy hair. The time to moisturize the scalp is in the shower, immediately after shampooing, when you can rinse any

excess conditioner out of the hair. If a dry-scalp condition persists, consult a dermatologist, who can prescribe a product to treat the extreme scalp dehydration.

Note: Your scalp may become dry at any time of year because of perming or coloring. If you develop a scalp problem soon after having your hair colored or permed—or performing either of these chemical processes yourself at home—it is a good idea to bring the problem to a dermatologist's attention, as it may be the result of an allergy to or irritation from one of the chemical ingredients. Don't let the fact that this is not your first use of the particular hair color, body wave, or perming product fool you: Allergies are by definition adverse reactions to ingredients that the body has come into contact with before.

THE SNOW-CAP
An Outdoor Activity Guide

The challenge that cold weather poses to a woman's skin is intensified by outdoor activity. Here are some quick tips for specific winter sports:

Walking or Hiking. In cold weather these activities can cause eyes to tear, lips to chap. The first course of defense: If it's sunny, wear sunglasses that block ultraviolet light. If you want to wear makeup, use waterproof mascara (which will not run down your cheeks if your eyes begin to tear) and a foundation formula that contains moisturizing ingredients to help buffer your skin against the cold.

Be aware that your lips are especially vulnerable to the elements because they contain no oil glands and are short on melanin, the skin's protective pigment substance (Don't let the darker color of lips fool you; the red tone you see comes from clusters of capillary blood vessels that are visible through the thin veil of lip tissue). Whenever you go outdoors in winter, apply a lip balm that contains both rich moisturizers *and* sunscreen ingredients (the same lip formula that you use in summer sun is one possibility but there are also products formulated specifically for snow and sun protection).

If you'll be outdoors for long and the sun is shining, be aware that snow can reflect a large percentage of the sun's rays back at your skin. Wear a sunscreen with an SPF 10 or 15—you'll still get some healthy color but you won't end up with a red, painful sunburn.

Skiing. As noted, this sport intensifies the "wind chill" factor of cold air against the skin. First, of course, protect yourself by dressing warmly in layers. Watch for exposed skin areas between the juncture of mittens and sleeves—you'll need thorough coverage if you don't want to end up with frostbite or red, wind-damaged skin.

Be aware that sun reflection can cause you to get burnt in unexpected spots—the sun will not only be beating down on you from above but bouncing up off the snow and hitting your body from below. Your neck, chin, eyelids, and ears will be especially vulnerable, so take steps to protect them. If you'll be out on the ski slopes for several hours, as most skiers are, carry sunscreen with you and reapply it at least every two hours—more frequently if your skin is fair or sunburn-prone.

Remember that lips need extra protection. While using the same lip moisturizer with sunscreen you apply in summer is one option, you might also want to look for a more emollient "glacier stick" lip protector, with extra moisturizer in the formula.

Don't neglect to wear sunglasses or ski goggles—and choose them not only for the color or design but for the amount of ultraviolet protection they provide. Squinting for hours on end increases the chance of developing wrinkles around your eyes at a young age—and the thinness of the skin around the eyes increases the potential for sun damage as well. If you prefer sunglasses, avoid those with metal frames, as they transmit cold back onto the skin. (See page 41 for further discussion.)

If your skin becomes very red or starts to burn, go inside quickly and *gradually* warm your body. (Don't make the mistake of going immediately from subfreezing temperatures outside to the hearth of a roaring fire: This increases the potential for skin "shock.") If your skin still looks very red and feels tingly, consult a dermatologist immediately, as you may have a slight case of frostbite, which can do long-term damage if it is not treated soon.

Sledding. This sport puts much of the same stress on skin as skiing. Along with the advice above, be sure to avoid staying outside if your clothes become very wet after you take several spills in the snow. To avoid frostbite or severe chapping, go indoors if you become soaked to the skin.

TWENTY HOT TIPS FOR WINTER BEAUTY

To help you look your best at this coldest, grayest season of the year,

I've assembled the following "hot tips" to keep your skin at its prime. Follow them and you'll see a definite improvement in the way you look this winter:

1. Practice "layering" of moisturizer, applying a first layer to damp skin, waiting five minutes, and applying another layer.

2. Carry a tube of hand cream in your purse and reapply it at regular intervals throughout the day, especially after washing your hands.

3. Never go outdoors in winter without wearing gloves. This will inevitably lead to dry, chapped hands.

4. Get a manicure regularly in wintertime, not just for the improved appearance of your nails but for the moisturizing benefits to cuticles and hands.

5. Avoid drinking alcoholic beverages before going outdoors into the cold, as this increases your chances of developing broken capillaries. In fact, you need to remember that while alcohol may seem to be heating up your body, it actually robs your body of natural heat. Sticking to hot chocolate or decaffeinated coffee or tea is a better idea.

6. Shampoo and condition your hair often in wintertime to offset scalp or hair dryness.

7. Try to perm or color your hair a little less often in wintertime—or practice preventive conditioning techniques. Every ten days, apply a mixture of one whole egg and half an eggshell full of olive oil to your hair before shampooing. Massage into hair and scalp; wait thirty minutes; shampoo and rinse twice.

8. Apply a rich moisturizing cream to hands and feet once a week, wrap in plastic bags, and wait fifteen minutes. When you remove the plastic bags, rub any excess moisturizer into the skin and wait a few minutes before getting dressed.

9. Be aware that the relaxing effects of a steam or sauna in wintertime can also be drying to the skin—a sauna more so than a steam bath. Limit your stay to less than five minutes, and never go into a sauna or steam bath that is heated to a temperature greater than 115 degrees Fahrenheit. Afterward, shower in warm water and slather on rich moisturizer from head to toe.

10. Switch to a milder skin cleansing routine in winter. Avoid toners that contain alcohol and use a rich cream cleanser that is appropriate for your skin type.

11. Before a bath, apply bath oil or high-quality olive oil to the skin. Wait one minute, then soak in the bath. This hot oil treatment should soothe tight, dry skin.

12. Avoid cosmetics that contain fragrance, as these also tend to contain an alcohol base that could be drying or irritating to your skin, especially if you are prone to dry skin at this time of year.

13. Continue getting regular salon facials all winter long, as they can help to boost your skin's moisture quotient considerably, especially if they begin with a gentle (not burning hot) steam treatment that returns precious moisture to the skin cells. (Avoid steaming your skin yourself at home, however, unless you follow the directions for home facials in chapter 2. Too-harsh steaming can do permanent damage to the skin.)

14. If you become tense during wintertime, it can take a toll on your skin. Try this gentle detensing facial massage: Apply a light moisturizer to

the face. With the palms of your hands, stroke your forehead gently from one temple to another. Use the same movement from chin to temples, then from the corners of the jawbone to the neck and shoulders. Repeat from the beginning, using slightly more pressure. Finish by shutting your eyes for a few moments. (This massage can be especially relaxing before bedtime.)

15. Spray a very light layer of hair spray onto your brush before using it, to avoid static electricity. And don't overbrush hair—it won't improve its appearance, contrary to myth, and can increase static electricity.

16. Use your blow dryer on the cool or medium setting rather than on the hottest setting, to avoid increasing scalp and hair dryness in winter, when the lack of moisture in the air will dry out hair and scalp on its own.

17. Apply a generous amount of cuticle cream or oil into the cuticle and nail area, and rub in with round movements of your thumb to help nail health and growth—and eliminate unattractive dry cuticles. Then soak fingertips in a bowl of warm water, to which you have added a little vegetable or bath oil. Wait five minutes, then rinse hands in clear warm water and apply a generous amount of hand cream.

18. Avoid nail strengthening products, especially those containing formaldehyde, as they can be extremely drying and damaging to nails and cuticles. Instead, get a professional manicure regularly and keep polish on nails all the time; these two steps will combine to eliminate nail brittleness and actually improve rather than damage nail condition.

19. Try the following soothing "eye pack" when your eyes become puffy or red from outdoor activities, such as skiing or sledding: Soak six teabags in boiling water. Allow to cool; when lukewarm, apply three to each closed eye. Wait two minutes; remove.

20. Use a night cream that is a richer version of the moisturizer you use during the day if your skin becomes dry at this time of year—even if you're in your twenties. To avoid getting cream on your pillowcase, apply night cream a half-hour before bedtime to allow it to soak into the skin.

BOTTOMS UP
Cold Weather Foot Care

When the weather is cold, we tend to bundle up—literally from our heads to our toes. It's not uncommon for our feet to spend all day in warm socks and even warmer boots, with the result being perspiration and, eventually, dry, irritated feet. The skin of our feet deserves special attention at this time of year, both to avoid unpleasant foot odor and to maintain smooth, unirritated skin.

The first step: cleansing the feet regularly and following every bath or shower with generous moisturizing of the skin of your feet. In the bath or shower, *gently* remove dead, flaky skin with the help of a pumice stone or skin brush. *Never* use a pumice stone or brush on skin that is not wet; it will lead inevitably to irritation and could even cause infection. Before putting on warm socks or boots, apply a perspiration-absorbing talcum powder to the feet; wait a few minutes before getting dressed.

One of the simplest ways to keep

your feet feeling and looking wonderful is to take advantage of professional pedicures regularly in wintertime. While most women tend to think of pedicures as a beauty service they get in the summertime, when strappy sandals and barefoot days at the shore put their feet on show, a professional pedicure can be an important *preventive* treatment in the winter, helping to avoid dry, irritated skin from appearing out in the open a few months later on. A properly done pedicure doesn't only include trimming of toenails and application of nail enamel; it begins with a skin-softening soak and includes generous moisturizing of the skin of the feet and gentle removal of dry, flaky skin. If you've no time for a professional pedicure, do remember to trim your toenails regularly to avoid ingrown toenails (always trim nails straight across). Follow these instructions for a foot-soothing treat:

• Fill a plastic tub with warm water and at least 1 cup of Epsom salts. Soak feet for fifteen minutes, then towel-dry.

• Holding your toes in one hand, bend and rotate your ankle inward and outward several times gently. Make a fist and massage the entire sole of your foot. Starting at the toes, take both hands and massage the foot gently, working back to the heel and up to the ankle. Repeat on other foot. Take each toe individually in your hand and pull it softly upward and twist slightly. To finish, massage your foot from the ankle to the big toe. Repeat on other foot.

• Next, use a pumice stone on the bottom of each foot to smooth calluses and get rid of dead skin. If the skin of the sides of your feet is dry, rub the pumice stone gently over these areas to remove dry, flaky skin.

• Apply a thick layer of rich, nonfragranced moisturizer lavishly over each foot up to the ankles. Wipe off excess around toenails and then weave a tissue in and out of toes.

• Trim and shape each nail into a neat square, using specially designed toenail clippers. *Don't* clip nails into a rounded shape; cutting them in at the sides can lead to ingrown toenails or infections. Simply clip them straight across and finish off any rough edges with an emery board.

• Stroke a base coat on each nail. Let dry. (You could use these few minutes to apply a rich moisturizing facial mask if you want to really treat yourself to a lavish at-home beauty treatment.)

• Apply a bright nail lacquer—for example, rich Christmas red, vivid hot pink, or shiny luminescent coral. Let dry; finish with a clear top coat.

For those times when you don't have the luxury of taking a half-hour out for a home pedicure, apply a homemade sloughing mask to the skin of your feet: Mix ½ cup sugar and ¾ cup sesame oil and apply to skin. Wait ten minutes; then slowly rub off the hardened mask in a gentle circular motion. Rinse with lukewarm water. Apply a rich moisturizing cream. Wait a few minutes before putting on socks or panty hose.

Should you use an antiperspirant spray on your feet? I don't think this is a good idea because it often leads to skin irritation and sometimes even allergic reactions. If you follow good skin hygiene and lavish a little attention on your feet, antiperspirant products shouldn't be needed. Better to use a lightly fragranced talcum powder on your feet than a potentially irritating chemical spray.

WINTER MAKEUP
Put on a Beautiful Face
❦

While a woman doesn't need a complete change in her makeup every season, she may want to reevaluate it and go for subtly different colors that will enhance the seasonal tone and texture of her skin. Many of the women who come to my salon complain to me about how dull and pale their skin looks in wintertime, and ask me what they can do to make their skin look healthier and brighter. The answer begins, of course, with taking care of your skin and keeping it in the best shape possible, avoiding the excessive dryness and flakiness that leads to a dull-looking complexion at any time of year. The other part of healthy-looking skin is using makeup in a way that enhances the look of your complexion, not by hiding it but by complementing it. (For complete, step-by-step makeup application advice, see chapter 15. This chapter also includes detailed information on choosing the proper makeup products and on getting the most from a professional makeup lesson.)

The key problem at this time of year is the fact that, for a Caucasian woman, wintertime means pale, sometimes lifeless-looking skin. When we are in our teens, our complexions maintain a pinkness and brightness during every season; once we get into our twenties, however, our skin begins to lose its youthful ruddiness gradually and to become a bit paler in cold weather. Moreover, we begin to spend less time outdoors. This is the time of year to choose a foundation that brings out the pink undertones of your skin—a foundation in a color that is *not* totally different from your natural skin tone (a clash between your natural color and your foundation equals unnatural-looking makeup) but that has a touch more pink in its coloration than the foundation you use at other times of year.

Remember that the impact of your makeup begins with the condition of your skin. Always begin with a cleansed "palette." This means gently cleansing your skin before every makeup application, using a liquid cleanser formulated for your skin type, and rinsing repeatedly with warm, then cool, clear water. Pat skin dry with a towel, then apply a moisturizer suited to your skin type (moisturizer not only sets up the skin for the application of foundation by smoothing it out and "filling in" any irregular patches but actually gives the makeup a better surface to adhere to, thus increasing how long your makeup will "last").

The cheek, eye, and lip makeup colors that look best in any season are, of course, those that are most flattering to your skin color and the colors that you enjoy wearing. In recent years, numerous so-called experts have come forward with strict color systems, specifying the precise makeup or fashion colors that a woman can wear and setting up rules for the exclusion of other colors. Many women who come to my salon for makeup lessons or application will begin by telling the makeup artist that they can wear only X and Y on their eyes and can never wear A and B lipsticks. When the makeup artist asks why they cannot wear such colors, their response often is: "I had my colors done and that's what I was told." Sometimes, women will even come into the salon equipped with swatches of the colors that they "must" wear.

My—and my expert makeup artist's—response to these systems is that, while they may often be based on the logic of the artist's color wheel, they deny the fun and enjoyment that should always be a part of wearing makeup, especially in the winter season, when every woman feels her complexion and her spirits can use a little lift. A part of developing a sense of personal style is developing a knowledge of what you feel looks best on you, not only in terms of makeup but also in jewelry and fashion. Feeling comfortable with makeup means experimenting with different colors and methods of application. Many women are often surprised to find that the most flattering colors applied to their faces during a professional makeup lesson are exactly those colors that they never thought would work with their skin or hair color!

The place to start in deciding about makeup colors at this time of year is with colors that enhance how healthy a woman's skin appears. That usually means peachy or pinkish blusher colors; muted green, gray, and other deep-forest color eye shadows and liners; and ice creamy pastel–toned lip colors. In winter, I love the look of colorful mascaras—loden green, navy blue—that pick up, but don't overdo, the effect of eye liner in the same color shade. At every time of year, I think women should think in terms of makeup as enhancement, not cover-up; wearing too much makeup is not only old-fashioned, it is unflattering at every age, in every season.

What will help your makeup to look most flattering is the choice of tools you apply it with. It's worthwhile to invest in the best makeup sponges, brushes, and applicators that you can find—these will help you to apply your makeup more quickly and easily and to better effect.

If you feel your complexion really needs a lift at this time of year, you might want to consider having a professional makeup artist give you a lesson in applying the colors that will be most flattering to you. *Don't* make the mistake of loading on the blusher in an effort to give your cheeks a healthier glow; all that will happen is that your makeup will look obviously fake and overdone. A professional makeup artist can teach you how to choose the foundation color that will create the illusion of more skin color without looking unnatural. One expert tip for adding healthy color to your face: choosing a lip color in the pink or soft coral family that will reflect color back onto your skin. In winter, you might also want to layer a protective lip cream under your lipstick to keep your lips moist. If your lips become very chapped at this time of year, try to avoid wearing lipsticks that have a high fragrance content, as they can add to chapping. Instead, you might want to skip lipstick altogether on the weekends and apply a rich glacier stick containing emollients and protective sun- and wind-blocking ingredients until your lips are healed.

For *black women*, the same general rules about makeup choices and application outlined above apply. Black women do have one special concern, however: Their skin often becomes drier and has more ashiness during winter than at any other time of year, the reason that I recommend beginning makeup application with excellent skin treatment products. A moisturizer that helps skin to repair itself is a good idea at this time of year, as is a professional facial that boosts skin's moisture-retaining capacity and helps ward off excessive dryness. Choose a foundation that will help even out your skin tone, and blusher colors that have a soft pink undertone. Stay away from dark plum blushers or lip colors at this time of year, as they can actually drain skin of color rather than enhance your complexion. The most becoming shades for black women to wear at every time of year are those that tend toward orange—coral, tomato red, or red-orange. Berry or loden green eye colors are very flattering at this time of year; stay away from light blue or white eye shadows. As for lipstick, think in terms of bright corals or vivid orange-reds; if you want a subtler effect go for a softer pink or coral touched with a hint of gloss at the center of the lower lip (if you want to minimize lips slightly, skip the gloss). Avoid brownish lipsticks, as they can make lips and skin look dull. At night, if you want a bit more shine in your makeup, think in terms of a wonderful gilded highlighting powder, or a touch of glistening pink powder that has a bit of luminescence in the formula; avoid silver powders, as they tend to bring out the ashiness in a black woman's skin. The important rule: Use shine subtly, with the lightest of hands.

BEAUTY BOOSTERS
Coping with Holiday Overload

If the Christmas season rush often leaves you feeling less than sensational, it's time to start your holiday beauty preparations a little earlier this year. Improving how you feel, more and more studies show, actually improves how you look. Try to give yourself a bit of extra personal attention during the month before the holiday season—I promise it will improve the way you feel *and* look during the holidays:

• Start your day with breakfast. While that may sound like something that helps your stomach more than your appearance, researchers have learned that people who begin the day with breakfast (and *not* just a cup of coffee grabbed on the run) actually have more energy to spare throughout the day. And any woman who has ever looked at herself in the mirror when she feels fatigued knows that the look of energy is much more attractive than the look of exhaustion!

• Keep up your regular exercise program at this time of year. Not only will exercising help you to burn off calories (an essential for most women during this season of luscious temptations) but it can also have the wonderful side effect of enhancing circulation to the skin and boosting the look of a winter complexion.

• Take five minutes out of your day to do the following relaxing facial exercises: Start with a cleansed and moisturized face and a mirror that helps you see the movement of your facial muscles—and avoid furrowing your brow! Begin by doing some tension-relieving head rolls, slowly circling your head from front to back. To move the muscles of the entire face, say "I am bee-you-tee-ful" six times, making sure to exaggerate the vowels for a thorough stretch. Finally, purse your lips and fill your cheeks with air. Place three fingers on each cheek; push fingers in without letting air out. Hold for thirty seconds; slowly exhale. Close your eyes and breathe in and out slowly for several seconds.

• Rev up your skin's circulation and smoothness with a fifteen-minute towel-tent steam facial. Fill a pot with clear water, let it come to a boil, then take the pot off the stove and add lemon juice, a handful of chamomile flowers, or herbal tea leaves. Let the mixture steep for five to six minutes, then lean over the pot, keeping face at least 10 inches above the water and suspend a towel over your head to keep the steam flowing onto your face. Close your eyes; steam for no more than five minutes, taking minibreaks every one-and-a-half to two minutes. Rinse face with cool (not too cold) water and pat dry with a soft towel.

• Nourish dry skin with a facial mask made from ingredients found in your own kitchen: Cleanse face thoroughly, then apply avocado or sesame oil to your skin. Wait one to two minutes; remove excess oil with a pressed cotton pad. Rinse face with cool, clear water. If your skin is oily, substitute the following mixture: Mash a tomato with 1 tablespoon each honey, plain yogurt, and oatmeal. Apply to skin, avoiding area around the eyes, and wait ten minutes; massage into face gently; rinse off with cool, clear water.

• Treat your tired, red eyes to a relaxing treatment: Brew six tea bags in boiling water. Let cool by placing mixture in the refrigerator for a half-hour. Apply three teabags to each closed eye. Wait ten minutes; remove; rinse eyes with cool water. Or, as an alternative, cut two slices of cucumber and apply each to closed eyes. Relax, put your feet up, and wait fifteen minutes before removing.

QUESTIONS OF THE SEASON

Q: My skin looks so washed-out in winter. How can I enhance it with makeup without looking overly made-up in outdoor and indoor winter light?

A: Just because the weather is gray doesn't mean your skin has to look that way. A little makeup know-how can transform your looks and warm up a winter pallor.

One option: Dust a pink-toned blusher (never a too-dark or too-brown shade, which looks unnatural) along your jawline, under your chin, and down your neck. When light hits it, the pink will reflect upward to cast a bright yet subtle hint of color onto your face, warming up your complexion.

Another way to turn washed-out to warmed-up: Mix a dab of your summer bronzer with your moisturizer and use it instead of your regular foundation. *Don't* use bronzer alone at this time of year, however; it can be too intense and fake-looking on winter skin. The moisturizer is also needed to hydrate winter-dry skin. Another trick that will make you look as if you've just returned from a midwinter vacation: smoothing a sheer color wash (or color gel, as they're sometimes called) from your temples across cheekbones and on nose and ear lobes—the spots where the sun naturally hits skin. An alternative for oily skin: using a foundation that matches your skin, then whisking with a translucent powder a shade darker—or mixing a darker powder with an equal amount of translucent powder before applying to cheeks, temples, the bridge of the nose, and the center of the chin.

To make pale winter skin more attractive at night, try a trick that makeup artists often use: Choose blusher in a shimmery shade and sweep it across the top of your cheekbones, over the bridge of your nose, at the center of your chin. It will catch the light as you move, giving your complexion a radiance that mimics a sun-kissed flush.

One caveat about all of these makeup tricks: Use a light hand in applying color to pale winter skin. You'll want a hint of healthy color—not an obvious line of makeup.

Q: I know that using a moisturizer is important, but I don't understand how it works. Does it add moisture to the skin? What is the difference between formulas? What can a moisturizer do for my skin?

A: Moisturizing creams and lotions do not add moisture to the skin, but they do smooth skin temporarily by retarding moisture *loss* and helping the skin retain the moisture that it already has. This is why it is best to apply moisturizers to skin that is already damp; the principal way they work is to "lock in" the water present in the skin cells and prevent evaporation, an especial problem in dry, cold air.

Moisturizers come in two main forms—creams and lotions, both often containing special additives such as urea, lipids, and lactic acid that are naturally present in normal skin and are meant to increase the ability of skin to retain a high moisture content. Additives such as estrogen or other hormones, although they sound scientifically sophisticated, have few

real benefits. In many cases, all they do is cause a slight swelling in skin, which makes wrinkles appear temporarily less noticeable. Humectants such as glycerine have the ability to draw moisture into skin from the air; they are often included in many modern moisturizer formulas for this reason. Emollients work to soften the skin.

Cream moisturizers contain more oil than water and are therefore richer, more emollient, and more effective in the long run—the reason they are recommended for skin that is dry or prone to dryness, particularly in cold weather. Lotions, which contain more water and less oil, are lighter, and therefore usually recommended for skin that tends to be in the normal-to-oily range, or for dry skin in warm weather. (If your skin is especially oily or acne-prone, you'll probably still need a moisturizer but should look for one with a medicated, noncomedogenic— or non–skin-plugging—formula.)

The thinner one's skin, the more difficult it is to retain moisture within the cells. Everyone's skin becomes thinner with age *and* with the change to colder weather in winter. This seasonal change means that you may need to switch to a richer, creamier moisturizer at this time of year—or to use a richer moisturizer on sections of the face that become particularly dry. While a moisturizer on its own cannot keep skin from aging, it is true that the smoother the skin's surface, the younger it looks—and that using a moisturizer on a daily basis can create the illusion of younger skin as well as helping makeup to go on more smoothly. A moisturizer is an anti-aging beauty treatment, however, when it contains a sunscreen, a proven wrinkle-preventive ingredient. Use of one is advisable even in winter when you'll be spending a great deal of time outdoors.

Q: My chapped lips give lipstick an unattractive cracked look. How can I solve the problem and help my lipstick to last?

A: This is a classic winter problem—and one that, if it tends to recur year after year, should be treated by starting to prevent chapped lips early on, before the weather turns frigid. *Always* use a lip-conditioning stick or lip cream under your lipstick; apply it before any of your other makeup to allow it to penetrate the skin. Before applying lipstick, reapply lip conditioner, wait a few seconds, and blot off excess with a tissue. If you prefer using petroleum jelly on your lips, that is also fine—unless you begin to develop tiny bumps under the skin in the area right around your lips, as this indicates that the jelly is too "rich" for your skin.

To help lipstick last and achieve a professional-looking application, begin with a lip pencil—one that has been sharpened and then briefly rubbed on a sheet of paper to round off the point. The shade that works for just about everyone is beige with a touch of cinnamon or rose. Outline lips, then fill in with the pencil. Lipstick goes on top to add moisture and more color; while the lipstick will fade relatively fast, the pencil color underlying it will last much longer, with the result that your lips will never look bare. To cut down on chapping, reapply lip conditioner at midday, under and then over color. For lasting benefits, apply lip conditioner before going to bed every night in wintertime.

Q: I always develop dry, cracked hands in wintertime. What can I do to cure—and prevent—this?

A: Consider your hands—how much you use *and* abuse them. This, plus the fact that the skin of the back of the hands (unlike the skin of the palms) is not bound to ligaments and tendons, makes them particularly susceptible to the ravages of cold, dry air, indoor heat, and soap and water. In my salon, I see many women whose hands become so dry at this time of year that the skin literally cracks and bleeds.

Yet chapped hands are not inevitable in winter weather. The solution: Get into the habit of slathering on a rich hand cream or lotion (look for glycerine as one of the ingredients) every morning when you first wake up and before going to bed at night. Supplement this by carrying a tube of hand cream with you during the day (keeping one in your desk drawer is a good idea) and reapplying the cream at least once during the day. If your hands become particularly dry, apply hand cream generously before bed and sleep with white cotton gloves on—the heat will help the cream to penetrate, the gloves to keep the cream from rubbing off. Always reapply hand cream after washing your hands.

To protect hands from the onslaught of windy, cold winter weather, always wear gloves or mittens when heading outdoors at this time of year. And don't forget the rubber gloves when washing dishes or cleaning the house—they may look silly but they do help to protect hands from drying soap and cleansing agents. If your hands tend to perspire in rubber gloves, apply a layer of hand cream or lotion first, to protect the skin from the salts contained in perspiration.

If your hands have a tendency to be dry, try a weekly sloughing treatment, applying a cleansing scrub or grainy cleanser and rinsing with lukewarm water, following up with a generous application of hand cream. If you don't have a grainy cleanser handy, use oatmeal instead (not the quick version but the old-fashioned, whole-grained kind). Mash 1 cup of oatmeal in a blender until very fine. Place in a large bowl and rub your hands in the bowl, gently rubbing away dry skin areas. Rinse with cool water; pat dry; lavish on hand cream; wait two minutes; and apply more hand cream.

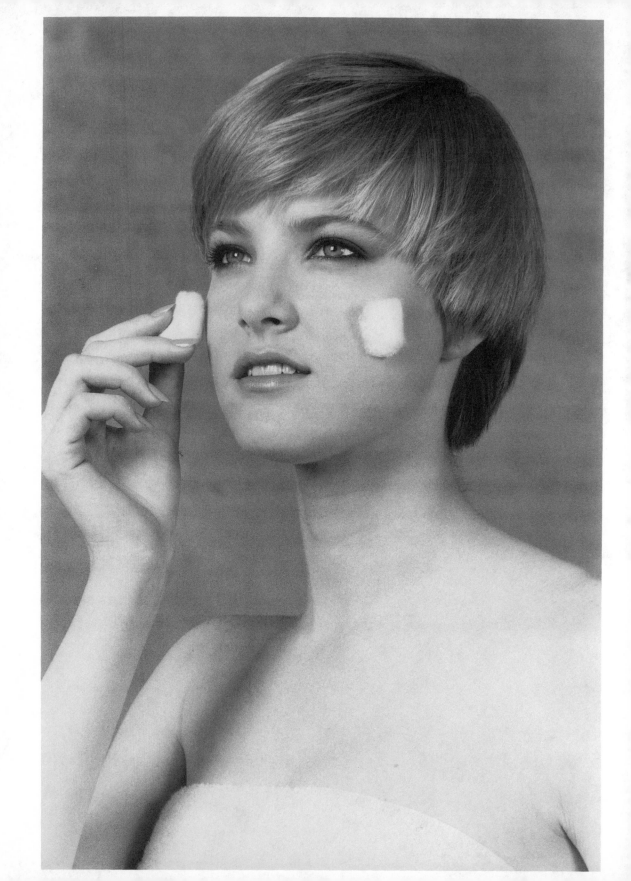

4

Spring Delights

Spring is a time of reawakening, of mild temperatures and clean, fresh air; it is the season that is kindest to the skin, as there are no extremes of cold or heat, dryness or humidity to add to complexion problems. The old custom of spring cleaning—of getting rid of the old and looking forward to the new—should not be a concept that we apply only to our closets. Spring is the perfect time to reevaluate your skin care routine, to pare down to the essentials and concentrate on making your skin healthy and attractive.

Each season has its own mood, its own look, so to speak. In springtime, every woman of every age wants her skin to look scrubbed-clean, fresh, full of life. This is the time of year to concentrate on your skin's condition, to do away with most of your makeup and go for a subtle, fresh-faced look. I'm not talking about going for the natural, no-makeup-at-all look on an everyday basis, but about really taking an honest look at your complexion and taking the time to care for your skin in the best possible manner.

THE PARING-DOWN PROCESS

The first step to better skin is to have your skin evaluated by a professional skin care expert. Even if you don't want to take the time or spend the money to have a professional facial (although this is the season when starting off with the benefits of a deep-cleansing facial makes real sense), I recommend that you do go for a professional skin consultation to discuss your usual skin care routine with an expert and learn how to have better-looking skin while spending less time caring for it.

Learning how to care for your skin begins with understanding its natural type—whether it is dry, oily, or a combination of the two—and learning about the kinds of products that will help keep your skin looking its best. Although understanding your skin type doesn't sound very complicated, many women do make mistakes. I have many clients who, for example, thought they had oily skin when in fact the surface shine was simply perspiration, not sebum (or the skin's natural oil). A woman whose skin is flaky, on the other hand, may have sensitive, oily skin and not a dry complexion. Too often, the products that we use on our skin actually end up camouflaging or affecting our skin type; a woman with a combination skin who uses harsh astringents, for example, may dry out her skin severely.

Whether or not you choose to consult a skin care professional, this is the time of year to concentrate on the old adage that "less is more." On weekends, try to wear as little makeup as possible; go outdoors wearing a sunscreen or moisturizer only, so that your skin gets a chance to breathe. Use a body brush *gently* while you're in the shower to remove dry skin from arms, legs, elbows, and knees. Add fresh vegetables and fruits back into your diet now that they are more readily available; a healthful diet can only benefit the appearance of your skin. If you have neglected exercising during the cold winter months—as we all tend to do—then take up the habit again: Go outside for walks, ride your bicycle, learn to play tennis if you don't know how already. Remember that all of the steps you take to improve the condition of your body will also benefit your skin; studies have shown that increasing circulation through exercise will also boost the circulation of nourishing body fluids to your complexion. The one caveat: Wear a sun-protecting moisturizer with an SPF 10 or 15 whenever you spend a good deal of time outdoors.

THE CLEANSING ESSENTIALS

In springtime—and at every time of year—the basis of good, clear skin is, first of all, skin that has been cleansed thoroughly and gently. When we are young, most of us use nothing more complicated than a bar of Ivory soap to wash the dirt and oil off of our faces and bodies. As we get older, we are struck by the multitude of choices, from soaps to cleansing bars to toners to masks, that are available merely for the purpose of cleansing the skin.

How do you know what to use? Depending on your skin type and your personal preference, you can clean and moisturize your skin with a variety of products. Here is a guide to making the right choices from the many options available today:

To take off your makeup—the first step to skin care of any kind, at home or in a skin care salon—the best thing to use is a creamy cleanser. Called "cold creams" in the past, these products are formulated to dissolve makeup, foundation, and lip and eye colors, and to make it easy to wipe them off of your skin. They are water-soluble, come in milky formulas, and are much gentler than a standard bar of soap. I myself don't use

soap and don't recommend it to my clients, as I feel that the detergent ingredients are too harsh for facial skin and can sometimes cause reactions in highly sensitive complexions. Another reason for my preference is that soap only cleans the outermost surface of skin, whereas creamy cleansers go a bit deeper, removing oil and makeup from within the pores.

To remove any cream residue it is then best to use a cleansing lotion in a formula that is appropriate to your skin type. The lotion should be of a high quality, with natural ingredients that nourish as well as clean the skin. Most cleansing lotions are clear liquids and are applied to the skin on a cotton ball; no cleansing lotion should ever be used near the eyes. I recommend that my clients go over their faces with a cleansing lotion twice to be sure that the skin is thoroughly cleansed.

To "wake up" your skin, the next step is to use a skin freshener, toner, or astringent. These three names, though interchangeable, usually signal products intended for different skin types. A freshener or toner is usually low in alcohol or alcohol-free and is intended for use on dry-to-normal complexions, while astringents, clarifying lotions, or refining lotions usually contain a higher proportion of alcohol and are intended for skin with a tendency to be oily. Wiped over freshly cleansed skin, these products restore the natural acid balance to the skin and remove any missed debris or residue left by soap or cleansing lotion. Astringents, by any of the other names, also impart a soothing, cooling sensation to the skin as well as the appearance of tightened pores (contrary to manufacturers' claims, no product can actually tighten pores, as the walls of pores have no muscles and cannot open and close like a door). Aluminum salts added to astringents irritate the skin slightly, causing it to swell and temporarily appear to have tighter pores. The principal ingredients in all of these products—astringents, fresheners, clarifiers, toners—are alcohol and water, in varying proportions. The products with the highest alcohol content are intended for oily skin, those with the lowest or none at all for dry or sensitive complexions. While studies show that the majority of consumers don't use astringents or toners, they are actually essential in cleansing your skin thoroughly, as they remove any traces of dirt or flakiness that can give the skin a grayish tinge. I recommend that all of my clients use a product appropriate to their skin types.

To maintain moisture in the skin, the next step is to apply a cream or lotion moisturizer (or day cream) to your skin while it is still slightly damp. If your skin is oily, you should use a moisturizer that is so light it absorbs into the skin instantly, with hardly any rubbing. If you have dry skin, you'll want to use a richer product that will provide more skin protection. Whatever your skin type, you should never apply makeup directly on bare skin, but should use a moisturizer as a buffer between skin and makeup. How to choose a moisturizer? Not by magical-sounding claims (which usually are not true) but by its texture, which can be easily tested in the palm of your hand. Another key point: A facial moisturizer should not be strongly scented, as fragrance ingredients can be irritating to sensitive facial skin.

To keep skin looking its best day

and night, every woman over age thirty should use a night cream, a richer moisturizer intended to safeguard skin's moisture balance while you sleep. If your complexion is very dry, you should use a nourishing night cream; if you have combination skin, a night cream should be applied to cheeks and under eyes only. If your skin is not wrinkled, overly dry, or flaky, you may want to use a night cream only every other night, so that you don't overclog your skin and encourage acne breakouts. An often-overlooked spot to apply night cream is the neck, often one of the first spots to "tell" your age.

To keep your skin looking young, the unacknowledged beauty essential is an eye cream. Starting in her twenties, every woman should apply eye cream twice a day, after cleansing her skin morning and night. The skin around the eyes is very thin, delicate, and lacking in oil glands, so it is the first area of the face to wrinkle or sag. Wearing a lightweight eye cream can help to protect this delicate skin and keep it looking young. The key to applying eye cream is to avoid stretching the skin around the eyes; pat the cream on, don't rub it in. Don't use an overly greasy eye cream, as it will tend to run into your eyes and cause them to tear and your eyelids to swell. Also, don't try to economize by using your facial moisturizer around your eyes, as most moisturizers contain ingredients that are too irritating for this delicate area. Also, eye cream should be applied so sparingly that it will last for a long time: Take a small amount of eye cream on the tip of your finger and pat it on under the lower lashes of your eye, from one end to the other, three or four times. Do the same on top of the eye, being even more sparing in the amount you apply. If your eye cream is so oily that it smudges your eye makeup in the day-time, it's too heavy, and you should choose a lighter, airier formula.

To enhance your skin's appearance once or twice a week, consider using a facial mask appropriate to your skin type. Masks—probably the least understood of skin care essentials—help to remove the film of dead cells, makeup, and oil that can often accumulate on your skin despite daily cleansing. Masks come in different categories for various skin types and contain natural ingredients that have been shown to be beneficial to the skin. For example, honey and milk are often used in dry-skin masks because they contain natural ingredients that can help to accelerate the blood—and moisture—supply to the complexion, while clay is a common ingredient in masks intended for use on oily skin because natural clay contains bentonite—a soft, porous, moisture- and oil-absorbing substance. Masks can come in powder, gel, cream, or paste formulas; the powders are mixed with water before they are applied, the others simply smoothed onto skin with fingertips or a minispatula. If your skin is dry, you'll want a mask that remains creamy while it is on; if your skin is oily, the appropriate mask to choose is one that hardens or shrinks as it stays in contact with the skin surface. This hardening doesn't tighten pores but does cool the surface of the skin as it dries it out. How often to use a mask depends on your skin's needs and your personal preference and time constraints, but no woman should use a mask more than twice a week. While using a mask sounds time-consuming, it takes a minute or two to apply, ten minutes to work,

and a minute or two to rinse off the face—not a lot of time considering both the real benefits that can be had, and the chance to take the ten minutes that the mask is on your face as relaxation time. Once important caveat: If a mask makes your skin feel irritated or itchy, or leaves it looking red, then the ingredients do not agree with your skin and you should not use the product again.

NATURE
Skin Nourishment

Once a woman understands the basic steps of skin care, the question arises not only of the types of products she should use but of which of the many legendary skin care ingredients are the best for her. In the last few years, skin care experts have frequently turned to nature as a source of skin tending and smoothing—and the number of skin care products that contain natural ingredients has multiplied. This does make sense, as, throughout history and around the world, women have used the essences of plants and foods to glorify their complexions.

How can a consumer tell whether a natural ingredient is necessary in a product—or whether it will benefit her skin? The first rule of thumb is to know your own complexion: If you have been sensitive to a given ingredient in the past, stay away from any new products containing that ingredient. If you have a tendency to be allergic to fragrances, flowers, or specific substances, read labels carefully to be sure that you do not use any products that contain these ingredients. If, on the other hand, you are like the vast majority of women and have been able to use cosmetics and skin care preparations with little or no problem in the past, then read on. I've chosen the most common ingredients and outlined the benefits and pleasures of their use in skin-care products.

Natural milk is commonly used in cleansing creams and moisturizers because it contains substances in the same concentration as our natural body fluids. Milk is very soothing and calming to the skin and can therefore be used on just about every type of complexion. It hydrates the skin naturally and contains proteins and sugars that help a moisturizer bind to the skin surface. In one Israeli chemist's research, it was revealed that milk contained nine different natural ingredients that could be beneficial to a woman's complexion: sugar to spur cell renewal; vitamins A and D to help prevent skin dehydration; vitamin B_1 to help regulate skin metabolism; vitamin B_2 to soothe skin; vitamin B_6 to help prevent pores from becoming clogged; vitamin C to act as a mild astringent; vitamin H to help prevent sunburn; and vitamin K to help strengthen capillary walls. Whether or not all of these claims are true, I have observed in my years as a skin care expert that the use of milk in various skin care products is very soothing to the skin and does seem to help replenish natural skin moisture.

Lemon juice is a common ingredient in astringents and toners because it helps to stimulate a tightening effect in the skin. In skin care preparations, the addition of a very small amount of lemon juice has a cooling and refreshing effect on the complexion; *never* apply straight lemon juice directly onto skin as it is too harsh and drying.

Yeast is a featured ingredient in many facial masks. It is a natural skin nourisher, helping to speed up cell respiration (or fueling) and to improve the appearance of every type of skin, especially skin with a tendency to be dry. Yeast masks are especially recommended for women whose skin is beginning to show the signs of aging.

Honey and *eggs* are often blended into masks and moisturizers for dry skin because they help to trap moisture within the skin cells and to accelerate the blood supply to the skin. Honey can also help to nourish the skin from the outside and acts as a slight antiseptic, or skin purifier.

Paraffin is often used as a final step in a salon facial or mask, as it helps to hold in body heat and speed the penetration of nourishing ingredients into the skin. Wax from natural sources is brushed onto a warm skin mask and left to set for ten minutes; it can also be used on hands as part of a manicure or on the feet as a final step in a moisturizing treatment. When the paraffin is taken off, skin feels noticeably smoother and softer.

Clay or mud are often used in masks for oily skin, as they help to absorb excess oil from skin's surface while soothing any irritated or blemished areas. Two thousand years ago, Israelis drew mud from the Dead Sea area to use in skin care preparations; today, many of the finest skin care lines still draw natural mud from this source. Natural mud contains potassium and sulfur in small amounts, which also help to clear a troubled or oily complexion.

Aloe vera is one of the most commonly found natural substances in skin creams and lotions. What is used is the aloe vera juice, or gel, derived from the spiny gray-green leaves of the aloe vera plant—a gel that has been used to treat burns (including sunburn), skin irritation, and even insect bites since the time of the pharaohs. Today, the aloe vera juice used in cosmetics is cultivated in Florida and southwest Texas. While experts debate the precise therapeutic qualities of aloe vera, many skin care experts concur that it does seem to have a soothing effect when applied to skin, and that it can be particularly beneficial to dry, chapped skin, whether due to sun or wind exposure. Many women like to use aloe vera skin care products in summer, too, because of the cooling feel of the gel against sun-warmed skin.

Jojoba oil, extracted from the peanut-size bean that grows on a spindly desert plant, is an ingredient that has gotten a lot of attention lately because of its ability to lubricate dry, parched skin. For more than four hundred years, Mexican women have been using jojoba oil as a skin and hair treatment. Today, jojoba oil is commonly added to hair conditioners, moisturizers, lip balms, and hand and body lotions in the United States.

Cocoa butter is frequently found in suntan preparations as well as body moisturizers. Derived from the roasted beans of the cacao tree, cocoa butter helps to lubricate and soothe dry skin and is a wonderful emollient in hand and body moisturizers.

Almond meal is frequently found in face and body scrubs, where it serves as a natural skin-buffing ingredient, helping to exfoliate dead cells from the skin's surface. The best almond meal is ground into a rounded, soft shape that gently exfoliates but does not irritate the skin.

Cucumber is a wonderful skin moisturizer and its juice is commonly used in alcohol-free skin fresheners meant to be applied to dry or sensitive skin. Cucumber is also a natural skin calmer and adds a wonderful fresh scent to skin cleansers and toners. Many skin care experts recommend applying a cool slice of cucumber to puffy eyes to eliminate skin swelling.

Whatever type of natural product you use, remember that the best natural ingredients are also those that are prone to rapid spoilage, so that all responsible manufacturers must include synthetic preservatives in their products in order for these preparations to last for more than a few days. In addition, just because a skin care product contains natural ingredients does not make it the best product on the market. Through trial and error, and the guidance of a skin care professional, you can find those cleansers, moisturizers, and masks that are right for your complexion and that are pleasant to use. At the first sign of any adverse reaction to a skin care preparation, consult a dermatologist or skin care expert, as you may be experiencing an allergy or sensitivity to a particular ingredient. If you are allergic to an ingredient, it is wise to find out which one, so you can avoid that ingredient in the future.

MASKS
More Than Skin Deep

I mentioned, in the step-by-step cleansing program above, that masks can refresh tired- or dull-looking skin by removing the dead cells from the surface. A mask can also provide a concentrated treatment for a particular skin problem, whether excessive oiliness, dryness, or sallowness. With the proper choice of ingredients, a mask can be formulated to rev up skin cell turnover, soften the skin, even out skin texture, or improve skin tone.

Whether to use a commercially prepared mask or to blend up your own skin potion at home is a personal choice; some women use homemade masks when they have the extra time to make them but rely on commercial formulas for their basic skin care regime. Masks made at home from fruits and vegetables cannot have the strength of commercial masks and are thus safe to use on an everyday basis; most store- or salon-bought masks, on the other hand, are formulated to be used once a week, every other week, or even once a month. A mask that you blend up at home will be completely natural, which also means that it will last no more than two days in the refrigerator before it will begin to lose its potency and to spoil. The results of using a natural mask are also short-lived, lasting a few hours at most.

Commercial formulations, however, are made with preservatives so that they can last six to seven months with refrigeration (I recommend that any mask, once opened, be kept in the refrigerator). Usually, the results of using such a mask can be seen on the skin for at least six days. Masks sold in a skin care salon will be prescribed for your skin by a professional, who can also advise you on how often to use the mask at home. A mask can be chosen according to skin type *and* desired effect—for example, a mask for dry skin that has a soothing effect versus a mask for dry skin that has a superhydrating effect.

The right mask can do more than improve the look and feeling of the outer surface of a woman's skin; it can also improve the look and feeling of her skin as it replenishes itself. A mask that fights oiliness, for example, can lessen skin oil output for days, not for merely that afternoon, whereas a moisturizing mask can allow a woman's skin to remain soft and smooth for a week, outlasting the effectiveness of even the richest moisturizer. All mask preparations are basically used in the same way, whatever your skin type or the mask formula you choose.

Applying a Mask

1. Remove all makeup with a creamy cleanser applied with a damp, clean cotton ball. Repeat until all traces of makeup are removed.

2. Cleanse the skin thoroughly with a mild cleansing lotion applied with damp cotton balls. Wipe repeatedly until cotton comes clean. Rinse with cool, clear water; pat face dry.

3. Dab eye cream around delicate eye area to moisturize during treatment. Masks should not be applied to the eye area.

4. Apply the mask preparation to the face with clean fingertips or a minispatula, excluding the delicate skin around the eyes. Only nonhardening (moisturizing) masks should be applied to the sensitive neck area.

5. Leave the mask on ten to twenty minutes (check the label if it's a store-brought product). Take this time to relax: Close your eyes, put your feet up, turn off most of the lights in the room, and put on soft music. A mask offers a psychological lift as well as a physical one, if you take the time to rest while the mask helps your skin.

6. Rinse your face with lukewarm

water; repeat until all traces of the mask are gone. Pat skin dry with a clean, soft towel.

7. Apply moisturizer, including on neck and eye area.

If you want to make your own springtime mask, here are some suggestions:

Peach Purée (for dry skin)

Purée 1 peach with skin (remove pit); mix with 5 pulverized almonds and 1 egg yolk. Apply to face, except around eye area (apply to neck area if you wish). Wait 15 minutes. Rinse face with warm water. Apply moisturizer and neck and eye cream.

Plum Perfect (for oily or acne-prone skin)

Boil 6 purple plums with skin approximately 10 minutes. Mash, removing pits. Add 1 teaspoon almond oil; blend well. Apply to face with fingertips or minispatula. Leave on for 10 minutes. Rinse with warm, then cool, water.

Mélange Mask (for all skin types)

Mix together 3 teaspoons beer, 1 teaspoon yogurt, $1/2$ teaspoon lemon juice, 2 teaspoons orange juice, 2 teaspoons grated carrot, and a few drops of olive oil. Apply to face with fingertips or a minispatula; leave on for 10 minutes. Rinse thoroughly with lukewarm water. Apply a lightweight moisturizer.

THE MAKEUP OF THE SEASON

At this time of year, most women want to use makeup to create a look of freshness; we think in terms of soft, rosy colors—pale pink, soft gold,

coral tones—added to the year-round neutrals to give skin more of a glow. Spending time outdoors on the weekends enhances skin circulation and texture, and a lighter feeling in clothes makes makeup less of an everyday necessity. Indeed, at this time of year, many women wear minimal makeup to work and none at all on the weekends.

The most attractive-looking makeup in spring, as in every season, is used to enhance a woman's features, not to hide them. With warm weather—and, sometimes, perspiration—here, it's wise to use a translucent powder as the finishing touch to your daytime makeup to keep shine under control. Here is a step-by-step guide to modern spring makeup:

1. Begin with clean skin. And remember, use a light hand to apply your makeup—strive for a sheerness of color, not an opaque cover.

2. Apply moisturizer only where you need it; apply eye cream around eyes.

3. Smooth on concealer, in stick or cream form, under eyes and anywhere your face casts a shadow. Dot on, then use a thin brush to blend. Start with a very light application; you can always add more if you need it, but it's hard to remove makeup neatly.

4. The next step is foundation, in a shade precisely matched to your skin. Some guidelines: If your skin has a yellow undertone, use a creamy, slightly yellow foundation (not one with rose tones, as it will clash with your natural coloring). If your skin is pinker, use a foundation with a bit of rose in the shade. Black women should stay away from foundations with grayish tones, as these tend to

emphasize any ashiness that may be present in the complexion; instead, look for a foundation that has a softness and pinkness in the color. Always match foundation to the skin of your neck. If you can't find a perfect match, buy two or three foundations and blend them together to create the right coloration. Use the palm of one hand as a palette to blend colors together before applying, beginning with the forehead, cheeks, nose, and chin. Blend the foundation out toward your ears and up toward your forehead. Then take a damp sponge and blot excess makeup away, using the sponge to blend into creases around the nose and any laugh lines around the eyes. Blend foundation slightly down the neck, so there is no sudden line at the jaw.

5. After waiting a few seconds for foundation to "set," apply blusher. Whether you use cream or powder blusher is a personal choice; women with very dry or wrinkled skin, however, should always use a cream formula. Choose a warm rose or coral shade; stay away from fuchsias or strong reds, as these tend to look brassy in the daytime under natural lighting. Find your cheekbones in the mirror by sucking in your cheeks, then apply blusher up the cheekbones toward the outer corner of your eyes. When you smile your blush should be on the "apple" in your cheek, but it should never be applied in a round shape, as this looks incredibly unnatural. Once you have brushed or patted on the blusher in the right place, use a fingertip or soft sponge to blend the blusher out into your foundation, so it is a soft hint of color, not an obvious stripe. There should not be any definite line of makeup on the cheeks (I emphasize this again as this is the most common makeup mistake and the one that looks most unattractive). You may also want to pat or brush on a bit of blusher around the forehead and on your nose or chin for a natural sun-tinged look. (If you use a powder blusher, then work with a soft, oversize natural-bristle brush to apply it in a soft sweep of color; then blend with a clean brush and set with translucent loose powder.)

6. For natural-looking eye makeup, use neutral tones, such as browns, grays, and taupe, touched with a hint of soft pink or yellow-gold in the springtime. Curl eyelashes first—this is a daytime substitute for mascara if your lashes are naturally full and long, and a good premascara preparation if your lashes need more help. For the softest result—what most women want in daytime, especially in spring's clear sunlight—use powder eye shadow, perhaps a subtle gray, applied all over the lid from lash edges to brow. (If your skin is very oily, apply concealer on lids first to keep shadow from creasing; if your skin is lined or creased, stay away from cream shadows, which tend to emphasize creases.) Use a soft natural-bristle brush to apply and blend the eye shadow, smoothing out any excess. Then, use a darker shade—chocolate brown or charcoal gray—to emphasize the shape of the eyes. Apply the darker color in a small triangle at the outer corners of the upper lids, then soften the result by brushing on a translucent powder shadow over the whole eye, in a shade such as soft pink or palest yellow-gold. If you want to apply eye liner, use a soft pencil that can be smudged easily, and subtly line upper and lower lids, then blend the color out. Finish with one or two coats of soft brown-black mascara.

7. In spring, lip colors can be softer, neutral, more natural looking. A touch of gloss as a finishing touch is another option for daytime. To give lips a neat look, line with a neutral lip pencil first, then fill in with a rosy pink, sheer coral, or soft taupe lip color, brushed on with a lip brush. Blot lips with a tissue for a matte finish. If you want a touch of shine to catch the sunlight, dab on a bit of sheer or taupe gloss in the center of the bottom lip.

T-ZONE CONTROL

With warmer weather comes the problem of avoiding the development of late-day shine—the result of perspiration or a bit of skin oiliness showing through sheer makeup and giving your face a shiny look. This usually occurs in the T-zone across the forehead and down the center of the face. While some women prefer the look of dewy makeup, no woman wants oiliness to upset the texture and finish of her makeup.

How to avoid late-day shine? By using the best possible skin care products to cleanse and prepare your skin before applying makeup. Begin by using a cleansing lotion formulated to control oiliness, then follow up with an astringent for oily skin. Don't make the mistake of thinking that pure alcohol would be the best oil-stripping astringent to use: While it is true that alcohol will initially strip skin of oil, it will spur a rebound effect of excessive oiliness. Instead, use an astringent in which alcohol is blended with ingredients such as sulfur, which will encourage long-term oil control. Once a week, use a clay mask to absorb excess oil and boost the effects of your skin care routine.

When choosing makeup, look for a foundation that contains as little moisturizer as possible. What you'll want is an emulsion formula that is high in water (*water-based* is the term most frequently used on labels) and that contains a bit of alcohol as well— a good choice is "pore minimizing foundation," as these are usually formulated for oily skin and contain a bit of oil-controlling powder. Before foundation, apply the lightest bit of moisture emulsion (a lightweight moisturizer for oily skin) to edges of cheeks, brow bones, edge of chin, or wherever skin tends to flake and become dry. Don't apply moisturizer where your skin is naturally oily (avoid nose, forehead, and center of chin), as this will encourage the development of late-day shininess.

As a final step, after you've applied all your makeup, use an oversize natural-bristle brush to apply a bit of translucent loose powder (don't choose a formula that is bolstered with moisturizer). Powder will not only help to set makeup; it will also act as a buffer against skin oiliness as the day goes on. In your purse, carry loose or pressed powder, which you can reapply in the afternoon to buffer your makeup further and help it to resist the absorption of skin oils. If your skin should become shiny, use a clean tissue to blot your face softly, then follow up with a brushing of loose translucent powder; this should not disturb the finish of your makeup but will cut down on skin oiliness.

POWDER VERSUS
CREAM MAKEUPS
Which to Choose

In warm weather, most women, whatever their skin type, like to use lighter-weight makeup formulas. Today, that doesn't only mean a choice between a liquid or cream foundation but can also mean an allover face powder. The choice of a foundation formula depends on several criteria: personal preference, ease of application, the condition of your skin, your skin type, and the effect you are after. How to make your choice?

Liquid Foundations. Usually the easiest for women to apply themselves liquid or lotion makeups come in a variety of formulas, from opaque to sheer, with a moisturizer or astringent base. The first priority is to look for the shade and formula that is right for your skin; in some cases, that may mean blending two colors together in the palm of your hand to come up with the perfect match (try to check a foundation shade on the skin of your neck whenever possible, not on your wrist; it is the contrast between a woman's makeup and the tone and texture of her neck that often makes foundation look unnatural). Women with very dry skin should look for a richer moisturizing foundation formula. The best way to apply a liquid foundation is as the professional makeup artists do: with a sponge. Apply a little bit of foundation first, then blend with a clean damp sponge, and reapply if necessary; it is always easier to add more makeup than it is to remove it midapplication. While it is most modern to wear a very sheer, translucent foundation formula, if your skin is blotchy or has areas of uneven pigmentation, it's best to go with a formula that provides a bit more coverage, or to use a heavier foundation as a base under a more translucent formula.

Cream Foundations. Cream foundations are the hands-down favorite of makeup artists because of their staying power—especially important under the hot lights in a photography, movie, or television studio. If you are not handy with makeup application, however, you may find that a cream foundation tends to streak or go on unevenly; try applying the foundation with a damp sponge, applying a little at a time and striving for the most even application. If your skin has a tendency to be oily or is prone to breakouts, it's a good idea to avoid cream-formula cosmetics, as they tend to be a bit heavier than other choices; for this reason, cream makeups are often preferred by women with dry complexions. Women with sensitive skin should probably not use a cream-formula foundation, though, as the more occlusive a product is, the more likely it is to irritate the complexion.

Loose Powders. Loose powders in soft pink, coral, or burnished brown can be used as allover face color in warm weather if your skin is smooth and blemish-free. Translucent powder has enough pigment to enhance skin and, if it is a high-quality powder, will have enough lasting power to keep a woman's makeup looking fresh all day long. For the most flattering effect, you'll want to choose a color of powder that enhances your skin, that has a bit more rosiness to it than most flesh-toned powders. The powder should be brushed on over moisturized skin with an oversize natural-bristle brush. If your skin has a tendency to become a bit shiny late in the day, look for a powder formulated to absorb oiliness—and freshen your powder at lunchtime. If you're concerned about blemishes, look for a powder that contains zinc oxide, which not only acts as a sunblock (a good idea for every woman) but is also soothing to sensitive skin.

QUESTIONS OF THE SEASON

Q: Help! I woke up this morning with an unattractive blemish and am scheduled to give a speech at work. How can I use makeup to cover up the blemish without its becoming more obvious?

A: First, make sure both your face and hands are clean when applying any makeup. Apply a very lightweight moisturizer to the rest of your skin (not on the blemish); wait a second or two for it to be absorbed into skin. Next, go over your entire face with foundation, using a small damp sponge to apply and blend. Then, "touch up" the blemish with a covering stick or cream perfectly matched to your foundation (the matchup between these products is essential for a natural-looking result, so you'll probably want to use concealer and foundation made by the same cosmetic company). Use a makeup brush or cotton swab to dot on concealer, then pat gently with the tip of the sponge to blend (don't rub, as this can irritate the blemished area). Two light applications are better than one heavy one, because you'll get a more natural, longer-lasting effect. To set your makeup, use a loose, translucent powder in an oil-absorbing formula. Use a cotton puff to apply powder with a gentle, patting motion, then dust off any excess with a clean puff or brush.

Q: Do I need to switch shampoos as the weather gets warmer?

What's the best way to find the shampoo that's right for me?

A: The only reason you'll need to switch shampoos in warm weather is if your scalp and hair usually become oilier at this time of year. In that case, you'll want to look for a shampoo that is labeled *for normal to oily hair*, which means that it has slight astringent qualities and will remove the oiliness thoroughly. A shampoo that contains keratin or protein will help to maintain a natural moisture balance in your hair, which is essential for its softness, luster, and manageability; a shampoo containing PABA will deposit a bit of sunscreen on the hair, a good idea to prevent the drying effects of everyday sun exposure (if you'll be spending a good deal of time outdoors, however, you'll want to use a sunscreening conditioner and a styling product that contains sunscreen, too, for the strongest protection against dryness and the bleaching of hair by the sun).

The only way to find the shampoo that's ideal for you is really through trial and error. One help is to discuss your hair type and needs with your hairstylist, who may be able to recommend a suitable formula. Bear in mind that we don't judge shampoos only by their formulation and cleansing abilities; most of us also prefer shampoos that have a pleasing but not too heavy scent and are either thick or liquid, depending on our own preference. The main ingredient in all shampoos is detergent, but the proportion of detergent to water and conditioning agents varies from one product to another and is not really listed on the label, although the ingredients are listed in descending order of concentration. (Because detergents may be listed by their complicated chemical names, however, ingredient listings are often of little help to shampoo consumers.) Some helpful shampoo-shopping hints:

• Start by trying a trial size of a new shampoo whenever possible. That way, if you really don't like the way a particular product works on your hair, you won't be stuck with a large bottle (how many half-used bottles of shampoo do you have lined up in your bathroom?).

• Choose a shampoo that cleanses your hair with one application. This is especially important if, like many active women, you shampoo your hair daily—and sometimes twice a day if you're exercising. Daily shampooers should never lather hair more than once, as too-frequent shampooing can dry out hair, leaving it brittle and lifeless.

• Never use a shampoo that leaves your scalp feeling itchy or irritated.

• Look for a shampoo that rinses out easily and doesn't leave any greasy or waxy residue.

• Don't judge a shampoo by its lathering abilities. Some manufacturers add foaming agents, which have no bearing on the shampoo's cleansing properties.

• Don't hesitate to alternate between different shampoo formulas. Switching off between a cleansing formula and a conditioning formula is an especially good idea, as it prevents hair from becoming too dry or developing a conditioner buildup.

Q: I usually spend more time outdoors in the springtime. Do I need a sunscreen, or can I wait till summer starts?

A: You definitely need to wear a sunscreen if you're spending time outdoors in the springtime. This is the time of year when the sun's ultraviolet rays begin to become more intense. The strength of sunlight—and its damage—is much greater on Memorial Day, for example, than on Labor Day weekend. I believe in going for the best protection against skin damage and aging possible: an SPF 15 sunscreen in a moisturizing formula, or, if your skin is particularly oily, in an astringent base. If you have fair skin, an SPF 15 will prevent your skin from burning, and should be reapplied often. If you have an olive complexion and want a bit of a golden tan, you can go to an SPF 10. Black women should not think that their skin's protection against burning is absolute, and should not face the sun without at least an SPF 4 or 6 at this time of year.

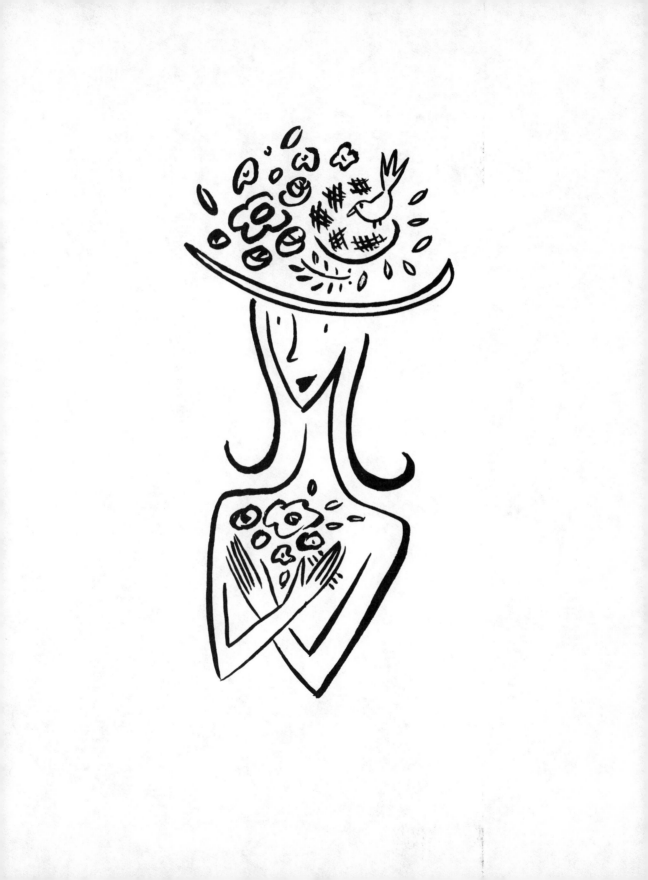

5

The Seasons of your life

We are all born with perfect skin—a fact every mother who has ever marveled at the smooth, downy-soft skin of a baby can attest to. The skin we are born with, however, is hardly the skin we keep; the marks and wrinkles of a life's experience eventually take their toll. The good news today is that, while it may be impossible to maintain babylike skin throughout a lifetime, a woman can take steps to keep her skin looking its best throughout her life.

In this chapter, I'm going to tell you how to do just that—how to have the skin you want, to make the most of your complexion at every age. Those women who maintain a youthful appearance throughout their lives often have the luck of good genes, but they also usually have the knowledge of skin care. And while my advice—and the best preventive steps—begin in childhood, I will also emphasize that good skin care can begin at *any* age. Of course, the best results will come to those women who start early, and to those lucky enough to have mothers who begin to educate them about the importance of skin protection and cleansing when they are young. Recent research shows, however, that even the most sun-damaged, sun-wrinkled complexion can begin to repair itself if a woman stays out of the sun, so the time to begin taking care of your skin is now.

THE SKIN OF OUR YOUTH

While I began this chapter talking about the perfection of a newborn baby's skin, it is also true that a baby's skin is fragile and sensitive and must be pampered to keep looking perfect. When a newborn leaves the protective environment of a mother's womb, the need for skin pampering begins. I myself was never so aware of this until I had a child of my own, and saw firsthand that a baby's skin could become as dry and irritated as any adult's.

Unlike adults, however, babies have complexions that give off very little natural oil; even a baby destined to become an oily-skinned teen will be likely to have dry, sensitive skin. The two skin care basics for infants are absorbing moisture from where it isn't wanted (on the outermost surface of the body) and keeping it where it is wanted (in the skin's lower layers). Cornstarch is still the best moisture-absorber to use on a baby's bottom (contrary to what most of us believe, talcum powder does not soak up wetness but actually causes it to bead up on the skin's surface). The best moisturizer for a baby's skin is a gentle formulation with a high lanolin content and a very low level of added fragrance (a probable skin irritant at every age). For very dry patches of skin, baby oil is a good choice.

Take care to protect your baby's complexion from the environment whenever you take him or her outdoors. Use clothes to keep wind and sun off the child's skin; bear in mind that the aging effects of sun exposure are cumulative, and that eventual damage can begin in infancy. While experts advise against using sunscreen on children under six months of age because the safety of these ingredients has never been tested on infants, it is important to protect even the youngest skin from sun exposure by covering exposed areas or keeping the child shaded if any time is to be spent outdoors.

From the time your child is six

months, be sure to use a gentle moisturizing cream and to clean the baby's skin with baby soap *only*. This is the time, too, to begin thinking about using a sunscreen on your child's skin (be sure to get your doctor's okay first, though, before applying this or similar products). Start to educate young children about the importance of cleansing their skin regularly (getting young boys to understand this is a real challenge!) and the wisdom of avoiding too much sun.

Throughout our childhood, we are pretty much freed from caring about our complexions, but it is a good idea to begin learning about the basics of skin care at a young age. While I don't recommend having a facial before age eleven, as the skin is too fragile (and even at eleven the most a young girl should have is a minifacial), I think it is not unwise to bring a young girl into a skin care salon for a consultation as soon as she expresses concern about her appearance. In my salon it is not uncommon for mothers to bring their nine- to eleven-year-old daughters to discuss wise skin care habits with me. I teach these young girls that the two most important steps to attractive skin are proper (not too harsh) skin cleansing and wise protection.

TEEN ANGELS

When I was a teenager, I didn't take kindly to advice from adults; I was as rebellious and stubborn as only a teenage girl can be. And lest any of my readers believe that this type of behavior is unique to American teens, I remind you that I grew up in Israel, a full two continents away.

The teen years are a time of rebellion, of finding ourselves and framing our identities—and the emotional turmoil of these years is often made worse by the appearance of skin troubles that threaten our already fragile self-images. An eminent dermatologist once noted that acne's impact was undoubtedly made worse by the way in which "our skin conspires to exhibit to the world around us the turmoil of our own emotions. As if being a teenager wasn't hard enough, having acne makes us even more self-conscious and self-deprecating than all teens already have the tendency to be."

But the fact is that having acne does not mean being powerless to improve your skin's appearance. The first rule of skin care to learn now: *Don't pick at your face.* Tiny scars you cause now can last forever—and become worse as your skin stretches and sags with age. What you *should* do is be as gentle as possible with your skin. Get a cleanser that is meant for oily and acne-prone skin and use it gently; rinse your skin repeatedly with warm, then cool, water after cleansing. Remember that acne is not caused by dirty skin, and can be made much worse by overzealous scrubbing or rubbing of the skin. If your skin is acne-prone, cleansing off excess oiliness can help to discourage future breakouts. Don't use a washcloth or loofah but *do* use a clean, damp cotton ball to apply cleansing lotion.

Keeping breakouts from becoming worse means doing as little as possible to your skin—not leaning your chin against the phone as you speak or cupping it in your hands during class (both common causes of later skin eruptions). It doesn't mean scrubbing at your face with harsh grainy cleansers, which can actually spread infection rather than help skin to clear up. If oil collects on your skin during the day, cleanse it off gently. I advise many teenage girls who come to my salon to carry cotton balls saturated with a low-alcohol toner in a plastic bag in their purse and to recleanse their skin at lunchtime in the bathroom at school.

If you wear your hair long—as many teenage girls do—try to keep it off of your face if you are prone to skin breakouts. Hair can spread more oil onto your skin, enhancing the chances for blackheads to form. If your skin is oily, shampoo it every day, and try to opt for a hairstyle that doesn't have bangs. Clean all of your brushes and combs by soaking them in a basin of water in which you have mixed a bit of shampoo once a week.

Other important steps to keep your skin looking its best at this age:

Keep your nails and hands clean. Not only do clean hands and nails look more attractive, they also help to prevent the spread of bacteria to your skin. The teen years are also a good time for a girl to get into the habit of grooming her hands and nails; well-kept nails are one of the details that are essential to a woman's attractiveness.

Treat a skin problem professionally when it's small. One mistake that many young girls make at the first sign of a pimple is to run to the drugstore and buy every possible skin cleanser, toner, astringent, and acne medicine they can find. Yet studies by doctors have revealed that *over*dosing your skin with many different medicated ingredients is more likely to cause skin irritation than it is to clear up breakouts. So avoid the temptation to use more rather than fewer skin lotions. Instead, consider having a consultation with a skin care

expert; even if you don't need a treatment in the salon, talking to a professional can give you the guidance you need to learn how to care for your skin at home. (Many salons offer consultations at no charge or for a nominal fee; call beforehand to check on an individual salon's policy.) If there aren't any skin care salons nearby, don't overlook complimentary consultations available at many department store cosmetic counters, or consider discussing your skin care purchases with the pharmacist at your local drugstore, who will have a great deal of information on the ingredients in over-the-counter medicated skin preparations.

Be aware of the diet-skin connection. While there are no magic foods that can guarantee clear skin (despite what the advertisements tell you), there is growing scientific evidence that eating a healthy, well-balanced diet can contribute to a sound, healthy body—including healthy-looking skin. Take time to eat real meals, not just snacks; the good eating habits that you develop now can stay with you a lifetime. After school, reach for fruit, cheese, and crackers, or a glass of milk and some graham crackers, rather than a bag of greasy potato chips and gooey pastries. Even though food oils don't literally "go to your skin," eating too much fat is bad for overall health, not to mention weight.

Don't fret over the inevitable skin changes that can come with the beginning of menstruation. It is a hormonal reality that a woman's skin can become oilier and more prone to breakouts at the time of her menstrual period. While there's no valid proof, many women insist that worrying about the look of their skin at this time seems to make it worse.

78

Don't worry. Instead, try to cleanse your skin more often—four times a day with a toner-soaked cotton ball carried in a plastic bag in your purse. If you can, take time once a week to use a clay-based mask; the natural clay in these formulas will help absorb excess skin oil. If your skin seems to become worse despite preventive measures, discuss the problem with a dermatologist or skin care professional.

Develop smart sun habits. While many young girls love to bake in the sun, science has proven that the suntan you get when you're young can contribute to skin aging and danger when you're older. I'm not suggesting that you give up the enjoyment of going to the beach and being outdoors with your friends in the summertime, but I do think you should learn to be smart about the sun. Use a sunscreen whenever you spend time outdoors in summer; consult the label of the product to see the SPF number that is appropriate to your skin type. If your skin is oily, don't use oil-based suntan lotions, as they can make your skin problem worse. Do cleanse off all sun lotions after you leave the beach by taking a bath or shower.

THE TREMENDOUS TWENTIES

The twenties can be the time of your life. This is when a young woman is graduated from college, begins to go out on her own, gets her first job and, often, her first apartment—in short, becomes more mature, more aware of herself and her identity.

This is also the time to develop adult skin care habits. At this age, it's a good idea to have your first consultation with a skin care professional if you haven't had one yet; this is especially true if, like many young women, you have moved to a city and are beginning to wear makeup every day. The combination of urban pollution and makeup often prompts the flare-up of skin troubles in the twenties.

At this age, all that most women need are "minifacials" done at home three times a week with a gentle grainy cleanser. Using this more efficient cleanser can help to sweep away remnants of makeup or dirt on the skin surface and help to keep your complexion smooth. I don't believe in using skin machines at home; they are usually too rough on delicate facial skin and can actually spread infection or irritation if a skin problem develops.

The twenties is also the time to begin thinking about preventing the wrinkles that can start to show in your thirties. This preventive care includes the following:

Always use a sunscreen when you spend time outdoors in summertime. Don't become frantic if you see your first laugh lines in the mirror, though. A face without any expression lines is very dull-looking and unattractive!

Be gentle with your skin. Use a sponge rather than your fingers to apply makeup, and avoid using harsh loofahs on your face (they're okay for body skin if yours is not sensitive). Always remove all of your makeup before exercising; if you don't, you'll only end up trapping perspiration onto your skin and encouraging breakouts or heat rashes.

Always shower and cleanse your skin immediately after exercising to ensure a smooth complexion. Perspiration that builds up on skin's surface can exacerbate a tendency to develop acne breakouts—a problem that by no means is limited to the teen years but can continue well into adulthood.

Get into the habit of using a moisturizing lotion on "quick-to-age" skin areas. These areas include the hands, neck, elbows, and edges of cheeks (the last is especially prone to dryness in wintertime, when harsh winds can be unusually hard on a fragile complexion).

THE THRILLING THIRTIES

Today, we think of a thirty-year-old woman as barely being an adult; she may have just gotten married and is more likely than ever to be a few years from starting a family. What a thirty-year-old woman should not be today is innocent about skin care. This is the time of life when invisible changes can take place beneath the skin surface that will make all the difference in how your skin ages; this is also the stage of life when skin protection becomes more essential than ever if you want to avoid as much skin sagging and wrinkling as possible later on. Some of the most important skin strategies for this stage of your life:

Cleanse your skin gently. Don't use harsh, grainy skin scrubs daily; being too rough with your skin can speed the breakdown of skin's supportive fibers (the most important precursor to skin wrinkling). Instead, use a gentle lotion-formula cleanser appropriate to your skin type (this is a key switch to make now if you haven't already) and, if your skin is oily, a gentle honey-almond scrub once a week.

Replenish skin moisture every day. In the thirties, the skin becomes less

able to hold onto moisture and needs more help in staving off evaporation from within cells near the skin surface. What to do? Always wear a moisturizer under your makeup, applied after cleansing, preferably when your complexion is still a bit damp (some dermatologists say you have three minutes after rinsing your face to put on moisturizer before evaporation begins in full force, so don't stall too long in the morning). Drink six to eight glasses of water daily and eat plenty of water-rich fruits and vegetables (cucumbers, lettuce, and celery, for example), avoiding such water-robbing dietary enemies as caffeine, alcohol, and sugar.

Let your skin "breathe" whenever possible. A healthy-looking complexion is not gotten by strangling your skin cells under heavy moisturizers and cosmetics on a constant basis. Always cleanse your makeup off completely *before* exercise class. *Never* sleep with makeup on. If you're heading for or living in a very hot, muggy climate, go light on your makeup, switching to water-based rather than oil-based formulas of foundation and moisturizer. Don't be so paranoid about the possibility of skin wrinkling that you overuse moisturizers; I see many women in their thirties who develop what I refer to as "aging-anxiety acne" caused by the use of antiwrinkling creams that are simply too heavy to be applied to young, basically healthy skin (not to mention women who, in their thirties, may still be prone to acne breakouts).

Protect your skin from the sun on a daily basis. If you wear a sheer foundation, don't rely on your makeup to accomplish this for you. Choose a moisturizer that contains sunscreen (an SPF 8 at least) and wear it every day all year round. In summer, switch to an SPF 15 on an everyday basis. If this sounds excessive to you, remember: Every bit of sun exposure is cumulative, adding to your risk not only of wrinkled, prematurely old skin but also of all forms of skin cancer. You can never be too protected from the harmful rays of the sun.

Start using an eye cream now if you haven't already. The thin skin around the eyes is the first to show signs of age, in the formation of laugh lines or crow's feet. While an eye cream cannot totally prevent this, it can make a difference in how obvious these lines are by temporarily plumping up the skin in this delicate area. One precaution: Don't overapply eye cream, as it will then seep into your eyes, where it can cause burning and itching at best, an allergic reaction at worst. To be on the safe side, if you have a history of skin reactions or allergies, opt for a hypoallergenic eye cream that is not overly greasy and is fragrance-free.

Take time out to pamper your skin. Women in Japan learn at an early age the relaxing benefits of gentle skin massage. This is the age when most of us can use the same special treatment. When applying moisturizer, take a minute to massage the skin gently with the pads of your fingers. At night, apply moisturizer to cheeks and neck in a gentle circular massage motion (your skin is still probably not in need of a heavy night cream at this age unless it is excessively dry). Invest in a humidifier to avoid the moisture-robbing effects of heated or air-conditioned homes. Don't wash your face in hot water; instead use complexion-pampering cool or lukewarm water.

Practice protective skin mainte-

nance, not just by moisturizing and sunscreening your skin, but by going for regular professional facials once every four to six weeks. The idea is to give your skin a gentle but thorough cleansing, and to apply protective nourishing creams. At this age, you should also have a professional skin care expert review your daily skin care routine to make sure that you are choosing the best skin care strategy for your complexion's needs.

Take care of your hands. Attractive hands mean more than well-groomed, polished nails, although they are undoubtedly important. What also counts is the condition, the smoothness, of the skin of your hands, which, like the skin of your face, naturally becomes a bit drier at this age. Always apply hand cream in the morning and before going to bed at night, as regularly as you brush your teeth. Then reapply it throughout the day if you have been outdoors or have washed your hands with soap and water. Avoid using harsh commercial soap formulas found in public restrooms whenever possible: They are meant for heavy-duty dirt removal and are not at all kind to your skin. When washing dishes or doing housework, wear rubber gloves (apply a layer of moisturizer underneath for a "minifacial" for your hands). If you are planning on doing some gardening, invest in a good pair of garden gloves to keep your hands from getting cut or pricked by stray brambles and to avoid the hyperpigmentation known as liver spots from starting to develop as a result of too much sun exposure. If you don't like wearing gloves, use a sunscreen lotion as a hand cream on days when you'll be spending time out in the garden.

THE FABULOUS FORTIES

As I write this, I have recently celebrated my own fortieth birthday (as well as the second birthday of my daughter, Segaal). I know that this is the decade when all of us, no matter how careful we have been to protect and replenish our skin, begin to worry about the subtle (and not so subtle) signs of age. A big difference today is that many forty-year-old women look far younger than their ages, and can keep looking good with proper care of their skin. The advice I give *and* follow at this wonderful stage of my life:

Stay under cover from the sun. As you know by now, this is my most important piece of skin care advice, but it is especially vital now, at an age when your skin has already begun to thin and to be much more vulnerable to assault. When we are young, we can damage our skin or neglect it and it has a remarkable ability to bounce back, but after forty, this is no longer the case. The sun exposure you get now will soon be translated into fine lines and age spots. Stock up now on sunscreens of SPF 15 and use them daily in summer; opt for under-makeup moisturizers, foundations, and lipsticks that not only contain skin emollients but are also high in sunscreens. Wear ultraviolet-screening sunglasses whenever you step out the door, summer, winter, spring, and fall. And always stay out of the sun during the peak damage hours of 10:00 to 2:00; do your outdoor relaxing, swimming, and tennis playing early in the morning or in the wonderful light of summer afternoons.

Be gentle with your skin. Even if you have always had oily skin, this is the age when you need to put away alcohol-containing toners and skin scrubs: They are simply too harsh for skin that is thinning and becoming delicate. Always wear a moisturizer, especially in winter. Get plenty of sleep and consider investing in a humidifier in your bedroom. Don't go to saunas or steam rooms for more than five minutes; they can sap your skin of "energy."

Be realistic; this is the best time of your life. I get very upset with clients of mine who are in their forties and fret over every single small line they see on their faces. At forty, a woman can be her own self, know her own mind, and look the best she has ever looked—but not if she is worried over every sign that she is no longer seventeen. This is not the age for even considering cosmetic surgery to make you look younger; it is simply not needed. What you need are good habits: Use sunscreen, get enough sleep, and do not overindulge in alcohol or drugs—and no cigarette smoking, which more and more research indicates cuts down greatly on circulation to the skin.

Be alert to changes in the texture or appearance of your skin. Some women find that their skin begins to change in their forties, and that the skin care products they have used for years are suddenly too harsh or too heavy. Along with regular monthly facials, a woman at this age needs to touch base with an expert every six months or so to be sure that her skin care habits are up-to-date and in line with her skin's needs. Often, women who have had oily skin their whole lives suddenly find that their skin "normalizes" in their early forties— and that the oil-stripping cleansers and water-based makeup they have been using for years are suddenly not right for their skin.

THE FANTASTIC FIFTIES AND SIXTIES

A woman who turns fifty can look in the mirror and see clearly the results of the care she has given her complexion, how well she has protected it against the ravages of sun, wind, and cold and whether or not she has given it the pampering it deserves. But even if you have been careless in the past you can improve the look of your skin at every age. Here's how:

Be gentle in skin caring. Use lotion-formula moisture-retaining skin cleansers and lukewarm or cool (not hot) water to wash your face every morning and night. Avoid skin toners containing alcohol, or grainy skin scrubs. When your skin needs extra care, whip up the following moisturizing mask: Grate raw beets and mix in a blender with sour cream. Apply to your face; lie down and relax for ten minutes. Rinse off with lukewarm water.

Stay out of the sun. This doesn't mean staying indoors but it means using full-spectrum (UVA- and UVB-screening) SPF 15 sunscreens and covering up with clothes in summertime. Suntanning parlors, harmful to skin at any age, are especially unkind to older skin, as it is more vulnerable to the insults of ultraviolet radiation (don't believe anyone who tells you that a particular suntan parlor is safe). Many dermatologists now feel that the lines and wrinkles that we associate with growing older are actually the result of "photoaging" or, more simply, having been out in the

sun! If you want to look as young as you feel, take wise steps to avoid getting too much sun.

Keep your body weight constant. An unfortunate fact of life is that skin no longer bounces (or shrinks) back very easily once a woman passes forty-five or fifty, so if you lose a sizable amount of weight later in life, you may find that your skin literally seems too big for your body or face. The wrinkles that seem to accompany weight loss are really the result of previously stretched skin.

Use moisturizers constantly. Don't let your skin confront the elements unprotected. Even if you choose to go without makeup on some days, don't go without a moisturizing lotion that is rich in skin-protecting emollients. And don't forget other weather-vulnerable areas, such as your hands, elbows, and legs (the last especially in summer). If your skin becomes very dry, mash half a banana with 6 drops of oil and 1 tablespoon of honey; apply to face, neck, and chest; wait five minutes; and rinse off in shower.

Remember that confidence and happiness are the best beauty builders. As we get older, it becomes clearer and clearer that a beautiful woman is a confident, happy woman who is at ease with her life. It is not something that comes in a bottle or jar with a magic gold lid, but a wonderful intangible that allows a woman to look her best at every stage of her life.

PREGNANCY AND SKIN CARE

The hormonal changes that take place during pregnancy affect the skin and hair in ways that can vary from woman to woman. For many women, bringing a baby into the world is the most positive, wonderful experience of their lives—so much so that they hardly notice the changes that take place in their appearance. I gave birth at the age of thirty-nine and found it a magical experience. Still, I continued to work hard in my salon, to exercise, and to live an active life almost up until my daughter was born. I found that my attitude counted for a great deal; I did not worry and just hoped for a healthy baby. I gained 45 pounds during my pregnancy, which is a little more than average. It took me seven to eight months to lose all the weight *plus* ten additional pounds that I had always wanted to be rid of!

For the first trimester, my complexion went through the worst changes—a problem that many women experience. My skin became flaky, dry, and itchy; other, especially younger, women often find that they develop acne blemishes and their skin becomes oilier than usual. Many dermatologists advise pregnant women to discontinue using all medications, including topical antibiotics. To cope with my dry, flaky skin I used a light peeling mask (available as a salon treatment or as a gentle exfoliating mask to use at home) and an oil treatment in the salon every other week. To deal with acne breakouts, a pregnant woman can have professional skin cleansing in a salon once a month or, if the condition is severe, see a dermatologist for more in-depth cleansing (don't try to treat acne at home, especially during pregnancy). If you have enjoyed steam rooms or saunas in the past, bear in mind that you should really avoid them now, as the stress to your body

of such extreme heat can be too much to take during pregnancy.

During the first three months of pregnancy, a woman's hair may also undergo some subtle changes. Mine became a bit drier, because my scalp was dry, so I used a conditioner more frequently and massaged the conditioner into my scalp for a few seconds before rinsing it out in the shower. One nice bonus of pregnancy is that a woman's hormonal shift will upset the usual shedding pattern of her hair, which means that you will hold onto individual hairs longer and shed less—making your hair look thicker than usual. This is especially nice if your hair tends to be fine and limp. After you give birth, the situation corrects itself, and some women fear that they are losing their hair; but within about six to eight months, the "catch-up" shedding ends and the prepregnancy hair thickness is restored.

The second trimester of pregnancy often brings with it a normalization of a woman's complexion and scalp. You may no longer need to condition your hair quite so often or to use an oil treatment on your skin. Stay out of the sun and have regular facials— they are as important to your spirits during pregnancy as they are at any other time, and offer busy women a good chance to relax. Try to avoid eating salty foods as much as possible; many women are especially prone to water retention during pregnancy. Regular pedicures and foot massage treatments can help to prevent swelling.

The last trimester is for many women the easiest. They have gotten used to the change in the shape of their bodies and are more willing to take it easy, perhaps because they become more excited with the approaching due date. I recommend to all my clients that they schedule regular salon facials, pedicures, and manicures during the last three months of pregnancy, as they will be so busy with a new baby afterward that they will have precious little time for themselves. I found that having regular foot and leg massages seemed to prevent the formation of varicose veins that so many pregnant women experience. In addition, being pampered was something I really appreciated having experienced during the first six months of my baby's life, when the only time I got to rest was when I was in my bed at midnight!

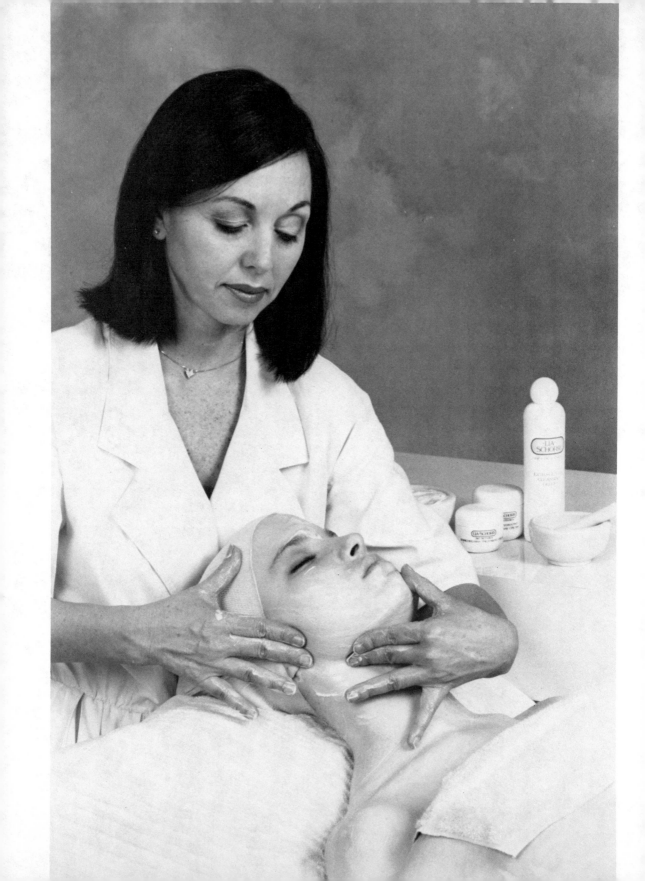

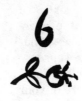

6

The Need
for Skin Care

Today, there is a great deal of attention paid to preventive health and fitness; but just as it makes sense to take care of your health, it also makes sense to take care of your skin, to help maintain its appearance and prevent the problems that can take their toll on your looks and your well-being. After all, just about everything that affects your mood or your health also affects your skin: What you eat; the climate you live in; whether your home is in a rural or urban area; the status of your marriage; your career; your age—all of these show up in the look of your skin. And while caring for your skin can't change the facts of your life—or your age—skin care can make a very real difference in the toll that time takes on your appearance. And scores of studies confirm that the better a woman looks, the better she feels about herself and the world around her.

Yet, for many women, the subject of skin care is scoffed at—or greeted with the question, "Who has time to use all those lotions and potions?" One of the first myths that I hope to have dispelled through this book, however, is that skin care must be complicated or time-consuming; in fact, skin care can be as simple or as involved as you want it to be. The choice is yours; and the role of a skin care expert like myself is to help you find the skin care regimen that not only works for your skin but that complements your life-style, your needs, and your image. What is also important is gaining a basic understanding of the structure of your skin, so that you can make sense out of all the skin care advice we are bombarded with these days.

SKIN STRUCTURE
Where It All Begins

The skin of the average adult covers approximately 18 square feet and weights an average of 6 pounds or more—making the skin the largest (and often least understood) organ of the body. The skin varies in thickness from the delicate skin of the eyelids to the more resilient soles of the feet and palms of the hands.

Every inch of skin contains millions of cells, along with sensory nerve endings and networks of vital blood vessels. The skin also is home to some 3 million tiny sweat glands that go to work when the body begins to register an increase in inner or outer heat. Each square inch of skin also contains a multitude of tiny hairs, many so fine that they can be seen only under a magnifying lens, others—as on the scalp—obvious to the unaided eye.

The skin is divided into three main layers, with the outermost, visible layer being the *epidermis*. The topmost portion of this visible layer is actually composed of dead skin cells that are continually in the process of flaking away and being replaced by new cells from underneath. When we are young and our skin is unscathed by age or environment, this replacement process is smooth; as we get older, this shedding, like all body functions, can become slower and sluggish and need assistance to be speeded up. Also within the epidermis are found the openings of the hair follicles and sweat glands commonly known as *pores*. The deepest layer of the epidermis is known as the *germinative* or *basal* layer; it is within this layer that new epidermal cells are formed and begin their journey upward to the outermost skin surface. In the epidermis are also found the skin cells that contain pigment (or melanin)—determinant not only of our skin's color but of our body's natural protection factor against some, but not all, of the hazards of the sun.

The second deepest skin layer is the *dermis*, which is primarily composed of the fibrous protein known as *collagen*, the same substance that gives skin its integrity, shape, and flexibility. *Elastin*, another substance important to the skin's resilience and youthful texture, is also concentrated within the dermal layer. When damaged by the sun's rays and the passage of time, the dermis begins to break down and stretch out, eventually forming the undersirable sags that show up on the skin's surface as lines and wrinkles. Within the dermis are also whole networks of blood vessels, nerves, and oil and sweat glands, as well as the "roots" of hair follicles. The nerve endings within the dermis are highly sophisticated; they are able to detect subtle differences in heat and cold, pain and pressure, vibration and movement.

The skin's innermost layer is known as the *subcutaneous tissue*. Composed primarily of fatty, or adipose, cells, this layer is the body's ultimate insulation and also gives the skin its smooth shape and contour. The amount of fat found in this layer, and its actual thickness, varies not only from one woman to the next but also changes from one part of the body to another—a result of body type as well as heredity. Age, sex, and general health all affect the fatty layer's thickness, but one thing is certain: If this fatty cushion becomes too thin, the body loses its ability to regulate its own temperature, to

function at a normal level, and to carry on regular body processes. While it may be true that a woman can never be too rich, as the saying goes, it is not true, from the standpoint of health and vitality, that she can never be too thin!

HORMONES
The Skin's Messenger System
❦

The pituitary gland—often called the master gland of the body's complex hormonal system—is a pea-size mass of cells attached to the base of the brain by a slender stalk of tissue. From this gland are secreted chemical messengers that control every body function from bone and muscle repair to body fluid balance to nervous-system reactions. Hormones literally determine how we act, think, and respond to the stresses of everyday life. The balance of hormones in our bodies controls our state of nervousness—our "fight or flight" responses—our moods, and, as a side effect, the health and appearance of our skin.

Hormones are one of the least understood factors in common skin problems, although they are believed by many medical experts to play a definite role in conditions ranging from acne to eczema to the growth of unwanted body hair. In the past, it was common to blame some skin problems in women on "an imbalance" of sex hormones; in fact, all of us—women and men—have both male and female hormones circulating in our bodies. The difference between the sexes is, in part, a result of the different proportions of these hormones, with women obviously having a greater amount of female hormones (such as estrogen and progesterone)

than of male hormones (testosterone and steroids). The latest theory concerning the causes of acne, in fact, is that certain differences within the skin itself can make some women especially sensitive to the *normal* amount of male hormones secreted by all of our bodies—so that what occurs is not an excess of male hormones but an oversensitivity to normal amounts.

In addition, many of the skin problems that are aggravated by tension—excessive skin oiliness *and* dryness—are believed to have hormonal connections, but this has not yet been proven scientifically. One thing is for certain: Skin changes such as breakouts that coincide with a woman's menstrual cycle or with pregnancy are also influenced by hormones.

Experts do not recommend, however, the use of skin care products containing human or animal hormonal extracts. In fact, many medical doctors feel that these products should be banned from sale, as their effects on the skin are unknown (many of these creams are imported from Europe and have not been adequately tested) and there are no proven benefits to compensate for possible dangers. Until more scientific information is available to confirm their benefits, these creams should be avoided. They are simply not worth the high cost, as they are not known to be any more beneficial than standard moisturizers.

SKIN TYPES
The Impact of Nature

The biologic structure of human skin is basically the same regardless of sex or race; but it is there that the similarities begin to dissolve. Our skin is, in many ways, a road map not merely

of our own contact with the environment but of our individual genetic histories. Granted, many of us reflect the influences of a melting pot heritage, but there are many remaining, and broader, genetic influences. In general, dermatologists divide skin into four main cultural types: white, black, Hispanic, and Oriental. Bear in mind that these are very general categorizations: Some factors within your category may not apply to you, or, if you are of mixed ethnic heritage, you may have influences from several different categories.

White Skin. This category actually falls into two basic subgroups: *fair* (Nordic/British) and *olive* (Mediterranean). Fair skin is light in color, thin in texture, and highly vulnerable to dryness, broken capillaries, and environmental damage due to sun and wind; fair skin is also more likely to be sensitive to ingredients, such as fragrances and alcohol, found in cosmetics. Olive skin tends to be oilier, more prone to blackheads and, by virtue of its darker pigment, better protected against sun- and windburn.

Black Skin. While its cells contain a higher concentration of pigment (melanin) than white skin, black skin is *not*—as many blacks erroneously perceive—immune to the hazards of sun-induced aging and skin cancer. Black skin needs protection, although it may not need the addition of heavy creams and oils.

A common misconception is that all black skin is oily. While the vast majority of blacks do have skin with a natural tendency to be oily, 5 percent of my black clients actually have extremely dry complexions, which often show up in ashy, gray-looking patches (these patches can show up on over-cleansed oily skin as well). Many black women also develop sensitivities to ingredients used in many cosmetics, or unknowingly induce skin breakouts by using heavy or greasy hairstyling products that accidentally get onto their skin.

Hispanic Skin. This type of skin is usually combination or oily—rarely dry. Hispanic women who have sensitive skin may find that a diet that reflects their cultural heritage (one that is rich in spicy or fried foods) can aggravate preexisting skin problems. While Hispanics tend to have olive-toned complexions that tan rather than burn when exposed to sunlight, their skin needs to be protected from the sun's damaging rays. It's not uncommon for Hispanic skin to have a tendency to scar after skin traumas such as acne.

Oriental Skin. This type of skin tends to have a smooth surface that, much like Oriental hair, beautifully reflects the light. What is also common among Orientals, though, is highly sensitive skin. Once it develops acne or blemishes, it tends to heal very slowly over periods of weeks rather than days—and is easily scarred if not cared for properly and allowed to heal gently.

Note: The darker your skin, the more you need to be aware of the possibilities of hyperpigmented (or dark-toned) scarring, and the more careful you must be to avoid self-treatment of acne blemishes. Just as your skin's melanocytes (or pigmenting cells) are better able to rush to the skin surface to protect your skin from sun damage, so too can they rush to protect your skin from other perceived attacks, such as the assault of squeez-

ing or picking at a blemish. The major consequence: Unlike a suntan, a pigmented scar will not fade away and, in fact, can grow more obvious over time. It is essential for every woman to resist the temptation to self-treat blemishes and acne breakouts, and to consult a physician or qualified skin care expert.

YOUR SKIN TYPE
Where Smart Care Begins

One of the basic questions that any woman concerned with her skin's appearance must answer is "What type of skin do I have?" While this sounds like a fairly straightforward question, I am continually surprised at how difficult it is for many women to answer. When women come to my salon, I routinely ask them during the prefacial consultation what type of skin they have. Answers range from "I think my skin is a little dry" to "I guess my skin is oily; I used to break out in my teens." What these answers tell me is that many women think they pay more attention to the condition of their skin than they actually do.

Knowing your skin type is not a one-time question; along with the change in seasons and age often come subtle or not-so-subtle changes in your skin's degree of oiliness, dryness, or sensitivity that should, in turn, signal a need for a different type of skin caring. Your skin is living, changing tissue—something too many of us tend to forget about, causing us harm in the long run. Continuing to use the same skin care products year after year because they were prescribed for you by a skin care expert ten years ago makes no sense at all; in fact, those products may be too harsh or too oil-laden for your skin's current condition, and can be the *cause* of skin care problems rather than the solution.

Whether your skin is oily, dry, or a combination of the two (as most women's skin tends to be) depends on many factors. Our skin is affected by the state of our health; by the environment we live in, indoors and outside; by the ratio of stress and relaxation in our life; by age; and by repeated sun or wind exposure. Just as you are probably not wearing the same clothes this month as you did a few months ago because the weather has changed, you may not be correct in thinking that you can use the same skin care products throughout every month of the year.

The best way to know your skin type is to have your skin analyzed by a skin care expert, who can then help you to tailor your daily and monthly skin care routine to your complexion's needs. But if you don't know of a skin care expert right now (more on solving this problem later), or simply want to satisfy your curiosity yourself, you can analyze your skin under an expert's guidance.

THE COTTON-BALL TEST

First, use this highly visual, simple test to get a general idea of your skin type. To begin, mix up the following tonic: In a blender, combine the juice of 1 lemon, ½ cup distilled water, 1 teaspoon of olive oil, and 3 ice cubes. Blend until the ice has melted. Then, brush your hair off your face (hold it back with a headband if it's long) and cleanse your skin using a gentle cleansing lotion (that's wiped off skin, not rinsed) rather than soap. Recleanse the skin with the tonic. Wait three hours. Then, wet three cotton balls with the tonic. Using a circular motion, gently wipe the first cotton ball across your forehead, the second down your nose, the third across one cheek. If all three come up clean, your skin is probably dry; if they're dark, it's oily; if they're slightly soiled, your skin, like most women's, is a combination of the two.

Now that you have a general idea of your skin type, it's time to take a closer look at your skin in a magnifying mirror. Choose a room that is brightly lit (near a window in daylight is the best; fluorescent light is the worst).

Look at your skin's surface. Are there uneven, flaky patches that seem to lift up from the surface? Do you see any red or parched-looking areas? These are signs of dry skin.

Examine your nose. Does it often look shiny within a few hours of cleansing? Do you see tiny blackheads, whiteheads, or skin eruptions? If so, your skin in this area is oily, a common condition even if the rest of your skin is dry.

Look at your hairline. Do you see any blemishes, blackheads, tiny bumps, or skin eruptions? These can be caused by excessive use of hair spray, gels, or pomades, or by perspiration or the styling of hair onto your forehead.

Focus for a minute on your chin. Look for bumps under the skin or tiny blackheads. Oily skin can be aggravated by bacteria or pressure coming from a telephone receiver or the palm of your hand, two unexpected but frequent causes of breakouts in the chin area.

Do you wear glasses? If you do on an everyday basis, take a closer look at the sides and bridge of your nose, where your glasses touch your skin. If you see tiny eruptions here, you may not be cleaning your glasses often enough—which should be, like your skin, a minimum of twice a day, morning and night.

Watch for these signs of skin that is sensitive. Whether your skin is dry, oily, or combination, look out for red blotches, broken capillaries, fine spidery lines, and isolated flakiness.

Don't be concerned if you don't especially like what you've just seen! I've yet to meet anyone, during all my years in the skin care business, who was 100 percent happy with the way her or his skin looked. Even those of us who are not at all concerned with our appearance will note the passage of time in our faces, will suddenly notice the results of one too many contacts with Mother Nature's extremes. Bear in mind, too: No one else looks at your skin through a magnifying glass, and for the most part, everything you are seeing right now can be improved with the help of the information I have given you in this book.

SKIN CARE
It's Logical!

Many women who have never been to a skin care expert dismiss the idea as something that is only for those who are rich, overpampered, or obsessed with their appearance. Nothing could be farther from the truth. From my experience, these women are not obsessed with their appearance or overly vain, but they do recognize that, in our modern world, how we look can affect our careers and our feelings about ourselves and other people. What a skin care expert offers them is expertise, the best possible skin caring, and advice on maintaining the look of their skin at home without using a lot of products or taking a great deal of time to fuss with their skin or makeup.

Another important factor in seeking out the expertise of a skin esthetician is that an expert can help you to *prevent* the majority of skin care problems. We can't stop aging but we can soften the effects that it takes on our skin; and we can also help you to weather the storms of changing climate, life changes, a new job, a new career, pregnancy, or divorce without having all the stresses of your life show up on your skin. Just as women today have learned that they can take responsibility, at least in part, for their own health, they are also learning that they can improve their skin's appearance by simple changes in habits (such as staying out of the sun) and routines.

One of the most frequent questions I am asked is "Why can't I just wash my face with soap and water, like I did as a child?" The answer is that while soap and water do work for some people, they don't work—and cause skin problems—for many adults. In all of my years as a skin care expert, the most appreciation I've gotten from clients is from those whom I have helped to find the proper cleansing routine for their skin type. Soap and water may leave your skin feeling superclean at the moment you use it, but it can contribute to problems ranging from tight, overdry complexions to oily residue that builds up to a shiny complexion by noon. Few women realize that a cleansing routine does more than remove dirt and excess oil from the skin's surface: It preps your skin for the challenges of the day, for makeup, for moisturizing, for facing the elements indoors and outside. Overcleansing or failing to cleanse your skin profoundly enough causes more skin problems than do any other skin care mistakes. Women who have sensitive skin, for example, often compound the problem by using too-harsh skin cleanser formulas. Ashy skin patches—a particular problem for black women—also commonly result from soaps that dry the skin; a change of facial and body cleansers plus a switch to a more penetrating moisturizer often clears up skin ashiness in a matter of days.

That doesn't mean, however, that a woman who comes to me for skin care advice will be handed a twenty-step cleansing routine involving a shelf full of products. In fact, I myself find many of the commercially available skin care lines to be too confusing, time-consuming, and unnecessarily complicated. I feel that any woman who is concerned about her skin's appearance need to start out with *just three skin care products: a cleansing lotion, a moisturizer* (both chosen for her individual skin type), and *an eye cream* (to help ward off one of the first facial "age zones"). These are the first three products I help my clients to choose. I advise them to use these products for several weeks, then to evaluate the impact they have had on their skin's texture, feeling, and appearance. Once many women see a visible improvement in their complexions, they ask me whether there are any other steps they should be taking to improve their skin further. It is at that point that I might recommend a creamy cleanser or makeup remover and a mask matched to their skin type, the last to be used once a week or every other week.

I am often asked about the multitude of other skin care products that are available at department store counters and in skin care salons. These products are all extras, not musts, and are meant for those of you who have a desire to take the extra time to make additional improvements in your skin's appearance. The idea that everyone who has an interest in looking better needs to start out with a list of products and steps several pages long is simply untrue—and reflects an effort of companies to sell products, not to offer true service to women and men.

Equally important to choosing skin care products is the results they provide—an area in which a skin care expert can offer a great deal more assistance than a department store sales clerk. If you don't see an improvement in your skin, or actually feel that it looks worse, then you can bring the problem to a skin care expert's attention. She or he should then evaluate your skin's condition and provide any replacement products at no additional charge. If you go to a department store to ask a question, you're not likely to get any help, unfortunately, aside from advice to buy another product. This is unavoidable, since companies are in the business of selling products rather than skin care services, as offered by a salon. In some cases, problems are caused by simply using a product incorrectly—either too often, or not often enough, or in the wrong amount—or by applying a product that is not right for your skin type or that is incompatible with other products you use.

GOING FOR A SKIN "CHECK-UP"

As a general rule, it's a good idea to check in with a skin care expert four times a year, at the start of each season, to reevaluate the products you are using on your skin and make a switch depending on the climate or the changing condition of your skin. In addition, I suggest that you consider visiting a different skin care salon, even just once, every few years, to see if there are new ideas that can be gleaned from a different expert, or a new type of approach that you might want to try. Even if you decide not to switch salons, you might come back with new questions, or new evidence that the skin care expert you have been consulting is the best for you. The same goes for your makeup artist and hairstylist; getting new input should not be taken as an insult to someone's service or expertise, but as an effort to supplement your beauty and skin care education.

PRO FACIALS
Skin Perfecting Plus Pampering

The essence of a top-notch facial is relaxed caring—a chance to feel pampered, to escape briefly from the pressures of a busy day, and to have your skin feel alive, refreshed, thoroughly cleansed and softened. To achieve all of this, the treatment must be customized to your skin's particular needs.

A proper facial takes about an hour—a little shorter if your skin is problem-free, a little longer if your skin is very clogged or has been neglected. Some salons offer what they call "minifacials," promising to have you in and out in less than a half-hour. I personally feel that in such a short time, a skin care expert cannot provide the combination of thorough skin care, advice for home caring, and skin information that a good facial should provide. The more a skin salon rushes the treatment, the

greater the chances of your skin becoming irritated or mistreated in the process.

A skin care specialist offers not only expertise but also the rare luxury of time for yourself. In a salon you are the focus of attention—very much a rarity today, when women often combine the roles of wife, mother, career woman, and active community member. While your skin is being cleansed and refreshed, you have time to clear your mind, gain perspective . . . even have a minivacation. (*Note:* There are some skin care problems a skin specialist should never treat, such as moles, severe acne, skin diseases, and rashes, all of which should be brought to a dermatologist's attention.)

Here, I would like to take you through my own personal version of a facial, explaining to you the purpose of each step, and why I believe that this type of facial combines the best of pampering and practical advice. This is information that can help you in choosing a skin care expert, wherever you live.

Step one: skin analysis. No facial should begin without a skin examination, first with the naked eye, then under a magnifying lamp. This skin "check" should be done on bare skin, from which all makeup has been gently removed. The analysis will take a little longer on your first visit, but should always be repeated on subsequent visits, as your skin can undergo changes—for the better or worse—between facials. The aim of subsequent analysis should also be for your skin care adviser to check whether your home skin care routine is working and whether it is helping to keep your skin in good condition. During the analysis, you should bring any problems that you have noticed to the expert's attention.

Step two: massage. As I said earlier, I believe that every facial should be relaxing, so the second step of every treatment should be a detensing massage. Depending on your skin type, this step may combine a neck and shoulder massage with a gentle facial massage. If your skin is acne-prone or very dry and delicate, the massage should be limited to the neck and shoulder area, since massage can aggravate acne or irritate very dry skin.

The relaxing effects are not limited to the area being massaged. Relieving stress from one area of the body has a wonderful carry-over effect on the rest of the body, spreading the relaxation benefits. A ten- to fifteen-minute massage can also help increase circulation, relax the muscles, and prepare your skin for the advantage of the skin benefits to come. Contrary to myth, massage, if done correctly, does not break down or harm the skin in any way. Our facial muscles are constantly at work, moving our faces into different expressions, helping us to smile, frown, and talk; gentle massage gives them a rest and increases your comfort in the salon and afterward. In fact, many of my clients tell me that the massage is the best part of their facials.

Step three: steaming. Using an aromatic mixture of herbs and soothing plant essences selected especially for your skin's condition, then blended into a warm spring-water infusion, the skin is steamed for about five minutes. This softens and soothes the skin. Steaming should never burn or irritate, and cool compresses should always be placed over the eyes first, to protect them. A vaporizing type of

machine is used to help control the temperature and intensity of the steam (this is much safer than simply placing a pot of hot water near the client's face) and it is also important that a rich cream be smoothed over the neck and left on during the facial.

Step four: cleansing. Once the skin has been softened, the skin care expert will cleanse the pores of oil and dirt, paying special attention to blackheads and whiteheads. An eye cream will be applied around the eyes, where no cleaning will be done unless absolutely necessary.

The cleansing should always be gentle. It should not be painful, although it may be a little uncomfortable if the pores are very clogged or if you have been ill or had a fever or never had a facial before—all of which can make the skin temporarily more sensitive. Always ask the esthetician to stop immediately if something hurts you; he or she may not be aware of how sensitive your skin is (although a knowledgeable expert should recognize this). Remember the facial is for you; anything that feels uncomfortable should be brought to the salon's attention.

Step five: antiseptic. The cleansing should be followed by the application of a soothing antiseptic lotion that tingles but does not burn.

Step six: twin masks. Two masks will then be applied, varying according to your skin type. The purpose of the masks is to complete the cleansing and soothing process, to help the skin recover and regain its "quiet."

The first "tightening mask" (so-called because it makes the skin feel a bit tighter and firmer) contains natural deep-sea mud, camphor, or soothing antiseptic herbs, depending on your skin's needs. It leaves the skin feeling refreshed and stimulated.

The second mask is a more nourishing, soothing, moisturizing mixture. It might be a honey and egg mixture or a fruit and vegetable mix blended with collagen and elastin moisturizers, depending on your skin type and moisturizing needs. Each mask is left on for several minutes (until it sets). It is removed with cotton dipped in natural spring water. The neck and eye cream is left on along with the mask, then the excess cleansed off along with the final mask.

Finishing touches. If this is your first facial and your skin is very dry and flaky, a light peeling mask may be applied to whisk away the dry skin cells that cause surface flakiness. Every facial finishes with a spray of skin freshener and a light moisturizer plus a final application of eye cream. Your skin should look radiant, glowing, refreshed—never irritated or blotchy—and your spirits should feel rejuvenated as well.

One final note: Many women who make appointments for a facial in the middle of the day ask to have makeup applied afterward. In my opinion, this is not the best idea, as the skin should be given a rest from any additional ingredients such as fragrance or preservatives after it has been thoroughly cleansed. Applying foundation, blusher, and face powder can be irritating immediately after a facial, especially if your skin has required profound cleansing. If you feel that you must wear makeup for a business meeting or appointment, I suggest using just eye and lip colors, as these two skin areas have not been manipulated during the facial.

SKIN CARE NO-NOS

It is important for any woman who is concerned with her skin's health and appearance to realize that all skin care experts are not equal. Always seek out a professional who has a solid reputation. Look for a specialist whose approach is informative, not pushy; you want information, not mere product sales talk. One factor that I cannot emphasize enough is the importance of personal rapport between you and the skin care salon staff. Look for a staff that is honest, warm, caring.

The atmosphere of the salon should be calm and peaceful, not like a huge sales bazaar. Beware of anyone who urges you to sign up for a series of treatments before you've even had a chance to evaluate the results of a single facial. While it is true that the care you give your skin needs to be done on a consistent basis, it is unfair to expect someone who has not had a single facial in a salon to purchase a series of four such treatments.

Some signs that a skin care salon is less than professional: if the massage is done after the cleansing (this can aggravate skin oiliness and cause postfacial breakouts); if your skin is very red and blotchy when you leave the salon; or if your skin feels irritated at any point during the facial. Remember, though, if you happen to have one bad experience with a salon, don't give up on professional skin care for good. As with any profession, there are good practitioners and bad practitioners working within the skin care field. In some states, skin care salons are required to be licensed, and this is a good starting point in evaluating someone's expertise; check with your local Department of Consumer Affairs (listed in the government-listings section of your telephone book) to learn what the laws are in your area.

A skin care salon that promises instant results is a sham. Just as skin irritations or eruptions don't develop overnight, they cannot be cured in a single facial. Each person's skin is different and takes its own time in healing itself. You cannot have skin like your neighbor's, your friend's, or someone you saw in the movies last night—even if you all go to the same skin care specialist! Don't be impatient. You will probably notice some improvement in your skin after a single treatment, but do not expect a complete change. If you have neglected your skin for years, you cannot expect a single visit to any salon to erase all of the damage. What a skin care salon *can* do is to make your skin cleaner and smoother, and to help it to look better and better as time goes on.

Another claim made by some salons that may not be able to be fulfilled is that they can make your skin younger overnight and take years off your appearance. My answer to this is that well-cared-for skin will always have the advantage of a youthful look and appearance. But there is no guarantee that going for regular facials will take any number of years off your looks. The biological age of our skin—as opposed to its chronological age—depends on a variety of factors, including genetics, the amount of sun exposure you have had in your life, your skin's dryness or oiliness (dryness tends to emphasize the obviousness of fine lines, oiliness to mask them), and the type and amount of makeup you wear. One of the most important services a skin care expert can offer is to help you to choose the right products to emphasize your skin's youthful glow—and to learn to use sunscreens regularly and liberally, because sun protection is the

only true anti-aging product that exists for the skin.

Above all, a skin care professional can also help a woman to cultivate a positive attitude toward her appearance, to neglect the temptation to use more makeup as the years pass in an effort to hide the effects of life experience and the inevitable ticking of the biological clock. I tell my clients who are concerned about aging that the most important step they can take to look younger is to keep current—to wear their hair in a fashionable manner, dress conservatively but youthfully, and wear a minimum amount of makeup that flatters rather than hides their skin. After that, it's a matter of proper nutrition, exercise, good sleeping habits, and avoiding alcohol and cigarettes—because the same good habits that can help a woman's health are those that can help to safeguard a youthful appearance.

WHERE TO GO FOR THE BEST SKIN CARE IN THE UNITED STATES

Here is a guide to the salons that provide the most professional, personalized skin care treatments and advice across the country:

Lia Schorr Skin Care
686 Lexington Avenue
4th Floor
New York, NY 10022
(212) 486-9670

Aida Thibiant
449 North Canyon Drive
Beverly Hills, CA 90210
(213) 278-7565

La Belle
575 Sutter Street

San Francisco, CA 94102
(415) 433-7644

The Face Place
339 Kearny Street
San Francisco, CA 94108
(415) 781-8153

The Face Place
2203 Chestnut Street
San Francisco, CA 94123
(415) 567-1173

Leah Kovitz
New Image
8391 E. Hillwood Lane
Tucson, AZ 85715
(602) 298-5801

Georgette Klinger
Dallas Parkway
Dallas, TX 75240
(214) 385-9393

The Spa at the Crescent Salon
400 Crescent Court
Suite 100
Dallas, TX 75201
(214) 871-3232

Les Amis
168 Newbury Street
Boston, MA 02116
(617) 353-1981

Elodie Salon
5300 Wisconsin Avenue N.W.
Washington, DC 20015
(202) 686-9310

THE BEST SKIN CARE AROUND THE WORLD

Many women have found that part of
the pleasure of travel is trying out a
body-sloughing treatment, massage,
or thalasso-therapy (sea water treatment) at a spa (for a complete guide
to skin care while traveling, see chapter 16). Here is a list of some of the
most luxurious spas on the Conti-
nent:

Biotherm Deauville
Boulevard de la Mer
14800 Deauville, France
(tel.) 98-48-11

Grand Hôtel Beau Rivage
Hoheweg 211
2800 Interlaken, Switzerland
(tel.) 36-21-62-72

Grand Hotel de la Pace
3 via della Torretta
51016 Montecatini
Pistoria, Italy
(tel.) 758-01

Hotel Bristol
3954 Leukerbad
Vallis, Switzerland
(tel.) 27-61-18-33

Orlane Beauty Institute
163 Avenue Victor Hugo
75016 Paris, France
(tel.) 47-04-65-00

Regina Isabella
Piazza S. Restituta
80070 Ischia, Italy
(tel.) 99-43-22

7

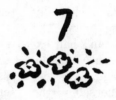

Great - Looking Hair

A woman's hair is literally her crowning glory. The look of a woman's hair expresses her sense of style, her self-image, the way she wants to present herself to the world around her. How many times have you felt dissatisfied with your appearance because you overslept in the morning and didn't have time to shampoo your hair—or because you've been so busy that you had to cancel your appointment for a haircut yet again? How a woman's hair looks often influences how she feels about her appearance to a far greater degree than any other aspect of her grooming. Yet having great-looking hair need not be difficult or time-consuming. What's required is a sense of style, of proportion, and a little bit of attention to caring for (shampooing, conditioning, and grooming) your hair.

THE PERFECT HAIRSTYLE

Every woman has had this experience: You walk out of a top salon, having spent a good deal of money on a new cut and style, and you couldn't be more disappointed. Your hair is not at all what you expected—it looks more suited to someone twice, or half, your age with absolutely different taste from your own!

I'm going to tell you here how to avoid that type of disappointment, how to communicate to a stylist what you want and—equally, if not more, important—how to select the stylist that's right for you.

Finding a stylist with a great reputation isn't hard. You can ask friends, relatives, associates at work; you can read magazines and newspapers and look for stylists who are called upon often by reporters for their professional opinions. You can even write to the beauty editor of a top national magazine to ask for names of one or two stylists considered the best in your area. But aside from reputation and technical ability, what most of us want is a stylist who has similar opinions about our hair as we do; even if we want a change in the look of our hair, we want the kind of change that is right for us.

How do you find out what a stylist is thinking *before* you get a haircut? Through a consultation. Just about every salon will be willing to grant you a consultation with a stylist, whether free or, more often, if the stylist has a national reputation, for a price. Even if the fee sounds high, pay it. A stylist may see you in short hair, and you may not want to part with your below-shoulder locks. If so, it's better to find this out *before* the stylist takes the scissors in his or her hands. At a consultation, ask questions—what type of style the stylist thinks would be most flattering to you, and why; what you can do to make it easier to style your hair at home; how often you'll need to trim your hair as well as to get a haircut; whether the stylist feels your hair color needs any help, or whether you might benefit from a body wave or perm; and how the stylist can help to improve your hair's condition. Be honest with yourself about your hair, your face, your appearance. If you bring photographs of styles you like, don't choose those that are completely opposite to what you have now. If you are five feet tall and have curly brown hair and deep-set eyes, bringing a picture of a 6-foot tall blonde with stick-straight hair and huge baby blue eyes is simply asking for the impossible—which is not what a beauty salon can give you.

At the best salons, your consultation will take place while you're in your street clothes; the stylist will ask you to stand up, perhaps even to walk up and down the aisle of the salon. Don't be surprised—your hairstyle should work with your life-style, your self-image, and the way you present yourself. Expect the stylist to ask you questions—about your life, your career, whether you exercise a great deal, whether you shampoo and blow-dry your hair every morning. Top stylists often ask about what's most important to you in a hairstyle to elicit your personal priorities. If a stylist doesn't ask you about something that you feel is important, volunteer the information. If the stylist is sensitive to the client's needs, you'll get feedback; if you don't, you probably should look for another stylist anyway.

What if you don't know what you want? If you have really come to the salon willing to be totally made over, then say it. But say it only if you really mean it. And be aware that allowing a stylist total freedom to do whatever he or she wants always involves a certain degree of risk, for you may not like what you end up with. The good part, of course, is that our hair is constantly growing, so it will be a matter of only two or three months before a given style grows out. (Of course, that isn't always much consolation if you truly don't like a hairstyle.)

After a consultation, the next step is an appointment for a cut. This appointment, too, should begin with a conversation, to see whether you've rethought any of the comments you made before—or whether you've had

a chance to see some other styles you like, either in magazines or on other women you know. This is your chance to say what you really want, so be specific. One way is to bring along pictures of the type of hair you want to have, whether photos of yourself in a past haircut you would like to try again, or magazine or newspaper pictures. Don't bring one single picture from a magazine, however; chances are you won't want a cut exactly like someone else's. You probably like the bangs of one cut, the length of another, perhaps the hair color of a third. A good stylist will be able to combine aspects of several hairstyles into one that works for you.

One of the often-ignored factors in getting the kind of hairstyle you want is listening carefully to what the stylist is telling you. Most good stylists begin by telling you a little bit of what they have in mind—and that is the best time to tell them if you disagree about any aspect of the cut. Don't wait until the cutting has already begun; a good haircut is a delicate balance of angles and lengths. Changing your mind midway may leave you with a less than perfect-looking haircut. What are some of the factors to consider in knowing whether a cut will be right for you?

Your personal preferences. For whatever reasons, most women fall into one of two groups: The "I like myself in long hair" group or the "I like myself in short hair" one. Even if the opposite is thought to be most flattering by others, we can't get away from our own opinions, our own self-images.

Your life-style—or the time factor. Twenty years ago, every well-

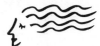

dressed, well-groomed woman went to the beauty parlor once a week; today, we not only don't call them *beauty parlors* anymore, we don't go nearly as often. If your schedule doesn't allow for more than a cut and blow-dry appointment every other month, then you won't want the kind of cut that needs continual fine tuning by a professional. If, on the other hand, your priority is always to have your hair looking its best and you will make time to get to the salon more often, then by all means let your stylist know. The same goes for hair color (which you'll be reading more about later in this chapter).

The "appropriateness" of a hairstyle. Even if we don't like it, we all have to admit that a woman who works for a Seventh Avenue clothing designer can probably get away with a cut that's a bit more trendy or avant-garde than a corporate lawyer or investment banker. Still, that doesn't mean that a woman who works in "blue-suit land" always has to have a conservative hairstyle. If you'd like the flexibility to have your hair look a little wilder on the weekends, then tell your stylist; today, a little mousse or gel and a blow dryer is all you need to change the look of your hair completely, if you know how. The best stylists will teach you how to change your hair when you want to, and will be sensitive to the demands of a career or lifestyle.

Your face shape, height, and features. The best-looking women have hairstyles that fit with the proportion of their bodies and their features. While it isn't necessarily true that only a tall woman can wear long hair, *how* long your hair stays should be influenced by your height, as well as by your posture and the way you

carry yourself. A good stylist will take all of this into account in discussing style options with a client.

THE SHAMPOO GAME

Today, the look of a woman's hair is as much a matter of its *condition* as of its cut. And the first step in hair care is the choice of a proper shampoo. The ideal shampoo cleanses hair gently, removing dirt, bacteria, and surface oils without stripping hair of essential moisture. This last factor is especially important today, when most women no longer wash their hair once or twice a week but *once or twice every day.*

The basic categories of shampoos are determined by hair type—dry, "normal," or oily. Recently, many hair care experts have stated that the last category, oily, is no longer applicable, as a woman who has oily hair and shampoos her hair every day would end up with dried-out frizzies if she used a very strong oil-stripping shampoo. Still, a woman who does a great deal of exercise—and perspires heavily—might want the extra cleansing power of a shampoo formulated for oily hair. Shampoo formulas that contain protein are especially common, and with good reason: Protein is a help to the appearance of damaged hair, which means hair that is frequently blow-dried, colored, permed, or abused by the elements. Protein deposits on the surface of the hair shaft make hair stronger and more resilient, as well as more manageable. (This tendency of protein to deposit on the hair shaft can be a negative factor, however, leading to shampoo buildup; if this occurs, ask your stylist to recommend a stripping shampoo, which should be used no more often than once a month to cleanse away excess conditioning deposits.)

The main ingredient in any shampoo is detergent, which loosens dirt and oil to cleanse the hair. However, the percentage of detergent in a shampoo varies from brand to brand, and there's no way of really knowing exactly how much detergent is present in a particular shampoo. Some preparations may contain too much detergent and be too harsh for your hair type. The best way to find out is to ask your stylist's advice. Otherwise, finding the right product is often a matter of trial and error. Experiment until you find a formula that leaves your hair soft, lustrous, and full of body. One way to avoid owning twenty-odd bottles of shampoo you don't like is to buy a small travel or trial size of a new shampoo, so you won't hesitate to throw out the remainder if you don't like the results after one or two uses. Don't judge a product by its lathering abilities: The amount of lather does not correlate with how well a product cleanses, as many manufacturers routinely add "foam builders" to their products that do nothing more than increase the lather without affecting the product's performance.

Many hair experts recommend "prerinsing" your hair before you shampoo by standing under the shower for thirty to sixty seconds to allow your hair to become thoroughly wet and enable you to use less shampoo. Whether the water is cold or warm doesn't really matter, but too-hot water can burn your scalp, so it should be avoided. Although the ability of a final cold-water rinse to "close the pores" of your scalp is legendary, there is no scientific basis for this. However, a cool-water rinse can be very refreshing, so long as you don't make the water *too* cold. Another help in cleansing your hair is never to apply the shampoo directly to your hair, where it will tend to pool in one area rather than spreading evenly throughout; instead, apply it to your hands and rub your hands together, then spread it into hair. Many women find that diluting the shampoo with a little water before applying it helps to spread it throughout the hair evenly. In any case, you should use as little shampoo as possible to avoid overdrying your hair; this is especially important if you shampoo daily—a practice that needn't be drying to your hair so long as you give it a single shampooing, a thorough rinse, and a gentle conditioning after every other shampoo.

Today, many of the best-selling shampoos contain natural or "botanical" ingredients. How do these benefit a woman's hair? Here is a fast rundown of the most common ingredients and how they affect hair's condition:

Aloe vera juice is derived from the leaves of the succulent aloe plant and has natural cleansing and moisturizing properties. Because of the gentleness of this ingredient, it is useful on all hair types. Aloe is also soothing to the scalp and mildly antiseptic, making it a good choice if your scalp has become sunburned or irritated.

Jojoba oil is extracted from the jojoba bean and was originally used as a beauty ingredient by native American women in the southwestern United States. Jojoba oil helps to add moisture to dry hair. Some women also find that a shampoo containing jojoba oil acts as a natural dandruff discourager, although it is not a medical treatment.

Natural henna is a conditioning,

rather than a coloring, agent when used in shampoos (check the label carefully, as some products found in health food stores may contain henna with its coloring ingredients left intact). Henna is of special benefit to normal and oily hair, imparting body and shine. Henna is also used in some shampoos for dull or damaged hair, as it can add shine, "strength," and manageability.

Vitamin E helps both to cleanse and condition hair, leaving hair with a glowing finish. In Israel, women pop open vitamin E capsules and mix them into commercial shampoos to increase the conditioning benefits.

Sea kelp is a natural source of collagen protein, iodine, and trace minerals, which help to condition the hair as it is cleansed.

Chamomile is found in many shampoos for blond hair, as it can help to bring out hair's natural sheen. It may also help to soften dry hair and increase its shine.

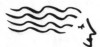

Balsam is an aromatic substance extracted from trees and shrubs that has conditioning properties for all hair types. It is often used in combination with keratin protein for enhanced conditioning effects.

SHAMPOO TACTICS

How to get the most from your shampoo? Not only by using the right product but by cleansing and rinsing hair well, bolstering the conditioning effects of shampooing with a gentle scalp massage. One of the reasons a professional shampooing in a hair salon is so pleasurable and effective is the scalp massage that accompanies the hair treatment. Here are simple directions for performing a relaxing scalp massage at home. Before you begin, be sure that your nails are trimmed and clean and remember to make all the movements *very* gentle:

1. Begin by brushing your hair vigorously for a minute or two—this acts as a gentle massage and also helps to bring the oils off the scalp and onto the hair, where they can be shampooed away (*always* wash your brush along with each shampoo to avoid redistributing oils and dirt back onto the hair later).

2. In the shower, wet hair well, then apply shampoo and work up a bit of a lather to distribute the shampoo throughout your hair.

3. Start at the forehead. Use your fingertips to massage the skin in a circular motion *gently*, working from the center of your forehead back to the temples. Repeat two or three times.

4. Place the fingers of one hand on the forehead, the fingers of the other hand on the back of the head. Using the pads of your fingertips, apply gentle pressure and move hands up and down. Repeat four or five times, changing hand position so that you massage your entire scalp.

5. Gently massage the scalp areas above both ears.

6. Using your fingertips, *gently* massage the back of your neck in a circular motion, then work forward to the crown and the front of your head.

7. Rinse well, then squeeze out excess water from hair and rinse again. Pat dry with a towel, then run a wide-tooth comb through your hair (don't brush hair when it's wet, as it is very vulnerable to breakage).

THE HAIR-DAMAGERS

Certain factors of modern life tend to rob hair of its shine and smoothness.

The first one is the daily use of a blow-dryer—which many of my clients tell me they couldn't live without. Perming, coloring, and straightening of hair, which can do wonders for the look of a hairstyle, are unfortunately also quite drying to the hair shaft. Heated rollers, curling irons, and heated styling brushes also rob hair of moisture and, when overused or used improperly, can lead to hair damage and breakage.

This is not to suggest that a woman must give up the convenience of hair appliances or the benefit to her appearance of hair color if she wants her hair to be shiny and healthy-looking. What is important, though, is to be as careful as possible in the use of styling tools and chemical treatments, so that you avoid the *unnecessary* hair damage that so many women mistakenly believe is inevitable. Some of the key steps to take to keep your hair looking its best:

Invest in high-quality hair tools. Combs and brushes of poor quality can literally tear at your hair, leading to hair breakage and damage. The best choice is a comb with rounded, even teeth that are widely spaced so that you don't catch at hair or irritate your scalp. A wooden comb is a good choice if you tend to have static electricity; otherwise, a hard plastic comb is a much better choice than metal, which can produce static electricity and is much more likely to have rough edges that can tear or damage hair. In brushes, the best choices are natural bristle or a blend of bristle and plastic; again, avoid inexpensive brushes with rough edges that can catch at hair strands. If you use a blow-dryer, always use a vent brush so that the heat of the dryer is not concentrated on scalp and hair. Choose a round brush for adding volume or turning hair under at the ends, a flat one for smoothing hair into a sleek shape. Experts note that brushes with rubber padding under the bristles are often gentler to scalp and hair, as the rubber pad absorbs some of the pressure during vigorous brushing. (Don't believe the old wives' tale of a hundred strokes a night, however; it's more likely to overstimulate the scalp's sebaceous glands and lead to oily hair than it is to improve hair's condition.)

Always blow-dry your hair on the lowest possible setting—and stop before your hair is bone-dry. Most of the damage that is done to hair by a blow-dryer is inflicted during the last few minutes of use, when some of the hairs are already dry and others are just a bit damp and the heated air removes every last drop of moisture from hair cells. A warm rather than hot setting is the best bet; if you finish with a cool blast of the dryer, your hair will keep its shape better during a minute or two of air-drying. When shopping for a blow dryer, stick with 800 to 1,000 watts of power and no more: A too-powerful dryer will lead you to inflict more damage on your hair than a slightly less powerful model. It's also a good idea always to hold the blow dryer about 6 inches away from the hair surface, so that the intensity of heat is lessened.

If you use hot rollers, choose those that provide "damp" styling. Dry heated rollers can rob hair of natural moisture; "wet-heat" rollers help to maintain hair's natural water balance. Hot rollers can provide some of the fastest restyling options, and are a good choice when you're going out at night and don't have time to shampoo your hair and start over. Never leave rollers in your hair longer than ten to fifteen minutes, and always allow hair to "cool down" for two minutes before unrolling and brushing out waves or curls.

Invest in professional hair color services. One of the top colorists in New York City has told me time and time again that he gained some of his most loyal clients when the women came to him to "rescue their hair" from hair-coloring disasters that occurred at home. Too often, the color that a woman sees on the box of home hair color is not at all the result that appears on her hair. A professional colorist can not only custom-blend a color product for your specific needs but also knows when to stop the coloring process to avoid hair breakage or overbleaching—the two most frequent reasons a woman who tries to color her hair at home runs to a pro for a "rescue."

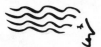

Be aware that illness and medications can affect the look of a woman's hair. Birth control pills, cortisone, sedatives, and thyroid medications all have the potential to precipitate hair and scalp problems. Not every woman will notice a change in the look or thickness of her hair while taking these medications but some will. Many women report that their hair looks thicker than ever during pregnancy, as the hormones released during pregnancy put a halt to the normal shedding cycle. Of course, our bodies "self-correct" after delivery, with the result that many women fear that they are losing their hair after giving birth, when in fact they are merely catching up to the normal hair-growth cycle.

Consult a professional if you are interested in perming or straighten-

ing your hair. The harsh chemicals used in perm and straightening solutions can wreak havoc on your hair's condition and seriously irritate your skin and your scalp. For this reason, it makes a good deal of sense to get a professional's advice before going ahead with these hair treatments, even if you still decide to do the procedure at home yourself. *Always* do a patch test first, applying the product to the skin of your arm and waiting twenty-four hours before going ahead with the perm or straightening process; if redness or irritation develops, don't use that product. Perm and straightener chemicals reshape the hair shaft by breaking down the chemical bonds, so use these products wisely; overuse, whether during a single treatment or by repeating the treatments too frequently, can cause hair damage and breakage. If you perm or straighten your hair, try to avoid blow-drying it, as it will be very vulnerable to dryness because of its weakened state. Try not to perm or straighten your hair more frequently than twice a year if you want to keep your hair in good shape.

Don't overuse styling aids, such as gels, mousses, and hair spray. These "liquid stylers" help to hold hair in place by forming a film on the surface of each hair shaft; over time, this film can build up, leaving hair dirty-looking, sticky, and dull. At that point, many women mistakenly believe that their hair is damaged and needs conditioning; adding conditioning on top of styler buildup only makes hair look even more limp and dull. The solution is to try to use as little mousse, gel, or spray as possible, and, if buildup has already occurred, to try one of the new "stripping" shampoos; these shampoos are supercleansers that remove conditioner and styler buildup and should be used no more often than every other week.

THE CONDITIONER CONUNDRUM

One glance at a shelf in a drugstore or supermarket and you can clearly see that there are conditioners for every possible need—protein conditioners, conditioners for permed hair, "extra body" conditioners, even, most recently, conditioners that promise to fight dandruff. There are instant conditioners, deep conditioners, conditioners meant to be used under a heated towel. Today, rather than suffering from hair in need of a conditioner, many women who come to my salon are actually *overconditioning* their hair; the result is limp, oily-looking hair that won't hold a wave or a shape.

How often should a woman condition her hair? It's a difficult question, depending on variables including how often you shampoo, the degree of damage you have already done to your hair, and the type of conditioner you use. Generally speaking, if you shampoo your hair daily (or, as many active, exercising women do, twice a day), you don't need to use a conditioner after every shampoo; that rule was developed, it turns out, when the average woman washed her hair once or, at most, twice a week. One problem today is that many of us still believe that we do need to use a conditioner after every shampooing, with the result that we are overcoating our hair with oil-based conditioning ingredients.

One of the side effects of overconditioning that many women don't realize is a tendency to develop acne along the edges of the scalp. Since conditioning ingredients are oil-based, when a woman perspires, a small bit of the conditioner often seeps off of hair onto the scalp and surrounding skin, where oily ingredients can clog the pores and lead to breakouts. The solution, it turns out, is simply switching to a "light"-formula conditioner and using it less often, say, after every other shampoo or, if your hair is in pretty good shape and you don't use a blow dryer every day, even after every third shampoo. One trend that is on your side is that conditioners have become more effective, meaning that they hold to hair better and do their job of softening and smoothing hair longer. Your hair may still look its best even if you use a conditioner no more than once or twice a week. (Another side effect of this improvement in conditioners, of course, is that the problems of overuse can occur even faster.)

What about "super" or "deep" conditioners? I recommend using these once a month, at most. They are usually so heavy that they can leave hair that is in good shape looking oily and limp. If you color, perm, or straighten your hair, then a deep-conditioning treatment, at home or in a salon, is a good idea once a month, as your hair will have a tendency to be dryer than normal. If your hair looks frazzled and flyaway, try mixing an egg or a bit of yogurt into your commercial conditioner to enhance its effectiveness.

WHAT ABOUT HENNA?

Pure henna powder has been used since Cleopatra's time to bring out red highlights in brown or almost-black hair. Today, it is used by many professional colorists as a natural alternative to peroxide in bringing out red highlights, and is also available for home use in powdered form.

The first thing to know about henna is that it acts as a permanent dye; although it washes out over time, the effects of henna can change the color of your hair for months, which means it shouldn't be used casually. The richness of the color that you get from using henna depends very much on the quality of the product; for this reason, I really think the ideal way to use henna is in a professional beauty salon. If you use henna at home, be aware that you may need to go through a little trial and error to get the precise effect you're after.

Begin by using as little henna powder as possible—you can always repeat the treatment but you can't undo the color once you've applied it. Start by doing a patch test, applying the henna paste to the inside crook of your elbow, waiting four hours, and examining the spot for redness; if the skin looks clear, wait another twenty-four hours and recheck the area. A lack of skin reaction after twenty-eight hours means you will probably be able to use henna without any problem (in some cases, however, you can get an allergic reaction to henna that is delayed until after you treat your hair a second or third time).

Don't use henna if you have already used a commercial hair dye in the recent past; any dye that is still on your hair can react with the henna and leave your hair looking bright orange-red—a not very attractive sight. Should your hair turn orange, you'll need a professional colorist's help in stripping your hair of color—and you'll also need to have him or her put color *back* into your hair once it's been bleached to almost-white. If you have naturally blond or light brown hair, stay away from henna; you'll

end up with vivid carrot orange stripes rather than highlights. Likewise, once you've applied henna, wait until it grows out completely before perming, straightening, or using other hair-coloring products on your hair, or you'll end up with disastrous results.

AT-HOME HELP FOR ADDING SHINE AND CONDITION TO HAIR

Many of the clients in my salon who love to make their own skin masks and cleansers have asked me whether I have similar recipes for improving their hair's sheen and fullness. To help them, I have developed a range of natural treatments that can be blended up at home with ingredients many of us already have on hand in our refrigerators and cupboards. Here are some of the treatments that have become favorites among my salon clientele:

Nourishing Shampoo
Blend ½ cup commercial moisturizing shampoo with ½ cup water (distilled if possible), ½ mashed avocado, and ½ cup regular shampoo. Use as you would a regular shampoo; rinse thoroughly with warm, then cool, water.

The Hair Pamperer
Mix together 1 whole egg, 1 teaspoon honey, and 2 tablespoons coconut oil. Apply to wet hair; leave on for 20 minutes (wrap hair in a warm towel while you wait). Rinse repeatedly with warm water; finish with a cool-water rinse.

Supersmooth Conditioner
In a small bowl, mix ½ cup coconut oil, 1 tablespoon eucalyptus oil, and the contents of 1 vitamin E capsule.

Comb through hair with a wide-tooth comb; wait 10 minutes. Rinse thoroughly with warm water; finish with a final cool rinse.

Hot Oil Treatment (for dry hair)
In a small pan, heat 1 cup olive oil until lukewarm. Remove from heat, test with a fingertip that oil is just warm, then apply to hair after shampooing. Put on a plastic shower cap (or wrap hair with plastic wrap) and relax for 20 minutes. Shampoo hair thoroughly; rinse repeatedly; shampoo again, and rinse repeatedly with warm water.

The Oil Beater (for oily hair)
Blend ½ cup white wine vinegar with ½ cup distilled water and 2 tablespoons chamomile flowers. Boil for 15 minutes, strain, then cool in the refrigerator overnight. Allow to come to room temperature, then use as a final postshampoo rinse to add shine to hair and discourage oiliness.

THE SHINE BUILDERS

The following recipes are for rinses that will help to bring out the natural highlights in a woman's hair. At the end of each recipe, I have listed a commercially available product that, while a bit less gentle to hair, can have similar results:

For Blondes Only
To bring out the shine in blond hair, use this rinse: Mix 1 tablespoon distilled white vinegar, the juice of ½ lemon, and 1 cup water (distilled if possible). After shampooing, comb the liquid through hair, then rinse out excess. (A commercial alternative: chamomile herbal shampoo.)

For Redheads Only
For fiery highlights, blend 3 ounces of fresh or frozen strawberries with 1 tablespoon red wine vinegar at high speed in a blender until liquid. Comb through hair after shampooing; wait 2 minutes; rinse repeatedly with warm, then cool, water. (A commercial alternative: Halsa Ginger Root Shampoo.)

For Light Brown Hair Only
For auburn and pale golden highlights, mix ½ cup plain yogurt with ½ cup blackstrap molasses and ¼ cup coffee grains. Mix thoroughly; comb through hair after shampooing. Wait 10 minutes, then rinse thoroughly with warm, then cool, water. (A commercial alternative to produce attractive highlights: Clairol's Summer Blonde.)

For Brunettes Only
A quick pickup for chestnut brown or deep black hair: Blend ½ cup molasses with 2 tablespoons of an instant conditioner in a blender at high speed. Apply to hair after shampooing; rinse out thoroughly with warm water after 10 minutes. Finish with a cool-water rinse. (A commercial alternative to bring out the natural highlights in your hair: Klorane Walnut Leaves shampoo.)

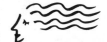

8

Hair Removal
- what's best

For many women—especially those of us who are brunettes or of southern European origin—unwanted hair is a real problem. Even blond women may be troubled by excess hair on their legs and underarms that they would like to remove. Today, there are a variety of hair-removal methods, temporary or permanent, that a woman can use. Some methods provide longer-lasting results than others—and some are better suited for use on specific body areas. In this chapter, I will give you the pros and cons of various methods—shaving, tweezing, bleaching, depilatory lotions, and electrolysis.

EXCESS HAIR
The Cause

Before a woman undertakes any type of hair removal, it is important to evaluate the cause of the problem. In most cases, it is merely a slight excess of hair that is an esthetic rather than medical problem; but in some cases, excess hair—or *hirsutism*, the medical term—has a serious underlying cause. A woman who finds, for example, that if she does not shave or bleach the hair on her face she would have a noticeable beard or mustache, might want to discuss the problem with a doctor, either a gynecologist or an endocrinologist, both of whom can tell by physical examination and laboratory tests whether the hirsutism is a sign of an underlying hormonal imbalance. If a medical problem is the cause, treatment with medications will help to halt the excess growth and a woman can then use hair-removal methods knowing that additional regrowth will not be as heavy.

One woman who came to my salon

for a waxing treatment was embarrassed to tell me that she had been shaving almost daily for over a year before she came to my salon; I noticed, however, that her hair growth seemed unexpectedly heavy. I suggested that she bring her problem to a doctor's attention. In a few months, she was taking medication that controlled her hair growth and was now able to have waxing treatments once every one or two months without the worry of heavy regrowth in between. While this may seem like a rare case, too many women fail to realize that excess hairiness can sometimes be a sign of an underlying medical problem, and that clearing up that problem can make any hair-removal treatment much more successful.

SHAVING
The First Assault

Shaving is the simplest form of hair removal—and one that, once a woman begins using, she usually has to keep up. Shaving removes hair at the skin's surface by literally cutting it off; regrowth is stubbly and rapid—so rapid that some women find that, to keep skin hair-free, they need to shave their legs as often as every day or two. Shaving is most suited, and most commonly used by women, for legs and underarms.

The best, most effective way to shave is when skin is wet and lubricated with a gel or cream. As dry hair can have the strength and stiffness of copper wire, make sure that hair is totally saturated with water before you shave. The ideal time to shave is during a shower or bath, and the ideal preparation is the application of a gel-formula shaving cream rather than a foaming product. Gels are the most concentrated form of lubrication and also best at providing a slick skin surface, so you avoid nicks and cuts. Don't shave right after you wake up in the morning; during sleep, body fluids pool in the legs and the skin swells, with the result that you won't get as close a shave at this time of day. Rinse your razor in hot water from time to time as you shave so that it doesn't get clogged, another cause of not-so-close shaves. If you use an electric shaver, make sure that hair *and* skin are thoroughly dry beforehand. An electric shaver does not give as close a shave as a blade, but it does have the advantage of not usually causing nicks and cuts, although it can irritate sensitive skin. Whatever type of blade you use, watch for the delicate underarm areas and along the bones of the ankles and knees.

Beware of chafing—dry, itchy, or bumpy skin—that can develop between the thighs or under the arms and is most commonly caused by razor irritation in winter, when skin is often drier and more sensitive. The solution can be to shave after you have been in the bath or shower for a while, when skin is more lubricated and less prone to irritation; don't use soap as a substitute for shaving cream, as it does not provide any skin protection. After you step out of the bath or shower, apply a generous amount of moisturizing cream and allow it to absorb into skin before you get dressed.

TWEEZING DOS AND DON'TS

Tweezing is a common hair-removal choice for eyebrows and stray facial hairs. It is an easy way to remove single hairs and "clean up" a facial area. While tweezing occasionally causes skin irritation between the brows, it is usually a temporary redness that disappears in a few minutes.

Always clean a skin area before tweezing with a mild cleansing lotion; and always flush with an antiseptic lotion and apply moisturizer after tweezing. Don't forget to sterilize tweezers with alcohol before using each time.

Beware of overtweezing eyebrows, which can produce a very unnatural-looking result. The idea is to maintain the natural shape of your brows and simply to "clean away" any stray hairs. If you find that you have a tendency to overtweeze, then consult a professional and have your brows done professionally once, watching how the tweezing process is conducted. Some women prefer to have their brows tweezed or waxed (see the section on waxing below) by a skin care professional at the same time that they have a facial.

If skin becomes very red or angry during tweezing, apply a drop of a calming facial mask, or blend a drop of chamomile powder into a teaspoon of buttermilk and apply. Yet another skin-calming option is to apply a cold sour cream or milk compress (a clean cotton ball soaked in sour cream or cool milk) to the skin area for a few minutes. (For more specific information on tweezing your eyebrows, see chapter 14.)

BLEACHING—HIGH CAMOUFLAGE

Many women find that bleaching the hairs on the face or forearms is a good way to camouflage unwanted hair without actually removing it. The results of bleaching usually last for several weeks at a time, and bleaching is easy for most women to do at home, using a commercial bleaching solution or a homemade version (see recipe below). *Note: Never* use any bleaching preparation on your face except those labeled *for facial use*, or severe reactions can occur.

Since it is not uncommon for bleaching solutions to cause irritation, it is wise to do a patch test before bleaching. Dermatologists actually suggest that this test be repeated before each bleaching session, as allergic reactions can occur at any time, regardless of how many times you have used bleach before. To do a skin test, blend up a small amount of the bleaching solution and apply it to the inner area of your forearm. Wipe away the solution but don't cleanse the skin with water or soap; wait one hour and check the area, then recheck for a reaction twenty-four hours later. If skin is not red, itchy, or irritated, you can use the solution.

The disadvantage of bleaching is that if you don't leave the solution on long enough—or fail to blend up a strong enough solution—the hair can turn orange rather than blond. The answer is usually to repeat the bleaching process until hair turns pale blond. *Never* use bleach on an irritated or broken skin area, as severe burning of the skin can result.

Another factor is that, while most young women's skin can tolerate bleaching solutions without severe problems resulting, it is very common for women who are over forty—and whose skin has developed a tendency to be dry and slightly thinner—to become irritated. If your skin is not sensitive, you can use the following bleaching solution after performing a patch test (see directions above):

Bleaching Solution

Blend 4 teaspoons lanolin with 2 teaspoons petroleum jelly, 1 ounce of 6 percent (or 20 volume) peroxide and 20 drops of ammonia. Apply to skin area, leave on for 2 minutes, and rinse off with cool-to-lukewarm water. Apply a gentle fragrance-free moisture cream to the skin area.

One important precaution: Never bleach your skin immediately before going out into the sun or into windy, cold weather, as irritation is more likely to develop.

WAXING
The Hows and Whys

An increasingly popular method of hair removal, waxing removes hairs slightly below the surface and encourages a softer, nonstubbly regrowth. Some women feel that, over time, waxing actually discourages hair's regrowth, but this has never been proven scientifically.

Waxing consists of melting specially prepared wax, cooling it to a comfortable temperature, and applying it to an area of skin; once the wax cools, it is pulled off against the direction of hair's growth and takes away the hair with it. Another variation is to use cold wax, though I myself feel that cold wax is not as effective and that it pulls harder at delicate skin areas, causing more irritation than benefit.

Used properly, waxing can keep skin hair-free for up to four weeks. Waxing can be used on the face, legs, and underarms. While it is often done at home, it is safest to have it done in a salon. Even in salons, a woman must be sure to check the technique that is used, to avoid skin irritation and allergic reactions.

There are two common methods of waxing: the European method and a more modern method. European machines use a solid block of wax that is melted under high temperatures; in some salons, after the wax is removed from the client's skin, it is redeposited in the machine, where it is melted and strained of hairs and then reused. While practitioners of this method claim that the high melting temperatures sterilize the wax mixture, I do not agree and feel that no woman should allow remelted wax to be used on her skin—I certainly would never agree to this method's being used on my skin. Hot wax strips, the modern method, are used once and then thrown away.

Even the most careful waxing is not without its possible side effects for women with highly sensitive skin. I feel that a test-waxing should always be done on the skin below the knees; if the wax causes redness or severe irritation, it should not be used and an alternative method of hair removal should be advised. Many women who can use wax without problems on their facial skin find that the bikini area is especially prone to irritation from waxing. It is also possible to develop a rash after a waxing, even if you have used the method without trouble for years. If slight redness develops after waxing, don't be alarmed; this type of reaction will clear up within ten to fifteen minutes.

Using wax at home is very common. The first caveat is to be sure that the wax is cooled to a touchable temperature before applying to the skin. It is not uncommon for me to see women in my salon who have burned areas of their skin after applying too-hot wax at home. Remember that while a burn heals over time, it always leaves a slight mark behind.

The proper way to apply wax, at home or in a salon, is to coat the skin with a bit of talc first, then to use a clean, fresh spatula to apply the wax in a room with good lighting. The wax should be allowed to cool to below skin temperature before it is removed by being pulled smoothly, in one direct tug, off of the skin against the direction of hair growth. (This last part, the smooth tug, is often difficult for a woman to do herself at home, as it is often slightly painful—and most of us have trouble inflicting pain on ourselves.)

In using wax in the bikini area, a woman or salon operator must be extremely careful not to apply the wax too close to the vaginal area, where severe irritation could result. Another factor important to waxing success is to avoid shaving in between waxings, as this makes the hair stronger and coarser, increasing the chances that post-waxing irritation will result. *Note:* Women who have varicose veins should never have their legs waxed, as this could aggravate the problem.

I myself have relied on waxing as a hair-removal method for the last fifteen years with a great deal of success and find that many of my salon clients agree. The investment of time in a salon is worthwhile, as the waxing is often less painful and the results last a month or longer, depending on the thickness of hair growth.

DEPILATORIES
Pros and Cons

Depilatories are a common hair-removal choice for legs, arms, and underarms; they should *never* be used on the face, where they can cause severe skin irritation, even on women whose complexions are usually not easily irritated.

Depilatory creams contain an active ingredient that chemically dissolves the hair above the skin line; this active ingredient is most commonly a form of thioglycolate—such as sodium thioglycolate or calcium thioglycolate—which is also the active ingredient in hair-straightening solutions. This ingredient, in high concentrations, melts away hair above the skin surface; it cannot penetrate below the surface and therefore provides results that last about the same amount of time as shaving, although regrowth is a bit less stubbly than when hair is removed with a blade.

Thioglycolate chemicals are necessarily strong—as evidenced by the often offensive smell of chemical depilatories (recently, some companies have introduced slightly better-smelling versions, but they are still far from pleasant). The presence of these chemicals on the skin for five to ten minutes—the time needed to remove hair—poses a problem for many women with sensitive skin. If you have ever developed a bumpy red rash after using a chemical depilatory, then you have had an irritant reaction to the thioglycolate ingredient. Because sensitivity can develop over time, you will notice that every package of depilatory cream or lotion contains the notice: "Irritation or allergic reaction may occur with some people, even after prior use without adverse effect. Test before each use by applying the product to a thumbnail sized area where hair is to be removed. Follow directions for use and wait 24 hours. If skin appears normal, proceed. Do not use on irritated, broken, or inflamed skin." *Always*

perform this test each time you use a chemical depilatory.

Always wait at least twenty-four hours before going out in the sun after using a depilatory. Regardless of how heavy your hair growth, never leave a depilatory on for longer than ten minutes; if all hair is not removed after this amount of time, repeat the depilatory treatment the next day. Be especially careful when removing hair in the bikini area to use a product that is labeled especially for bikini use—and keep the cream well away from the vaginal or perianal tissue, where severe skin redness and irritation can occur in a matter of seconds. To minimize the chance of skin reactions, look for a depilatory product that contains skin-soothing ingredients such as aloe, mineral oil, or lanolin. If a reaction occurs, rinse skin repeatedly with cool water and consult a physician as soon as possible.

ELECTROLYSIS
Permanently Hair-Free

Electrolysis is the only method of hair removal that is recognized as permanent by the American Medical Association. It is commonly used to remove hairs from the upper lip, chin, and bikini line; because of the time-consuming nature of the process, it is rarely used for large body areas. In the right hands, it can be a very rewarding treatment, freeing you from the worry of keeping skin hair-free; in the wrong hands, however, electrolysis can leave skin scarred, pitted, and irritated without satisfactorily removing hair.

The first step in considering electrolysis is to seek out a well-qualified practitioner; in states where electrologists are licensed, your task is made somewhat easier. In any case, your best bet is to ask a dermatologist for a recommendation. Because dermatologists often see the aftereffects of electrolysis at skin level, they are good judges of the quality and success of treatment. If you have a friend who has had satisfactory electrolysis treatment, ask her for the name of her practitioner.

Electrolysis consists of the insertion of a thin needle into the hair follicle and the passage of a mild electric current through that needle to remove hair at its growth source. Because every hair goes through a "dormant" as well as an "active" stage, no single treatment can remove all of the hairs in a given skin area; in fact, electrolysis usually requires several months to be effective. During your first visit with an electrologist, she or he should describe to you in detail what the treatment consists of and give you a rough estimate of how much time it will take to remove all of the hairs from a given body area. Even an area that seems as small as the upper lip may take months of treatments at roughly $60 each—a more expensive option than any of the temporary ways of hair removal, but a permanent one.

Done properly, electrolysis may leave the skin slightly red immediately after treatment, or even with a very small amount of scabbing. All marks or scabs should heal and disappear within a day or two, however. Any skin irritation, bump, or scab that lasts longer indicates improper treatment and should lead you to try another practitioner. Even the best practitioners cannot avoid causing a small amount of pain each time the needle is inserted into the hair follicle. Certain skin areas, such as the upper lip, are especially sensitive, and treatment is more painful. It is a good idea to follow any electrolysis treatment with the application of a gentle antiseptic and to wait at least an hour before applying makeup. Recently, because of scares about communicable diseases, many electrologists have begun to provide each client with their own personal electrolysis needles; the client brings the needles to each appointment and is responsible for sterilizing them between electrolysis sessions.

Even the most skilled electrologist will leave a woman with a certain percentage of what seems like regrowth. You should be aware that electrolysis only works on hairs present at the time of treatment; if excess hair is due to a medical condition, electrolysis will not affect the rate of future growth. Anyone who has a heart condition, who has a personal or family history of mitral valve prolapse, or who is prone to skin conditions such as eczema or psoriasis should not have electrolysis without checking with a physician beforehand.

Until recently, even electrologists were not that successful at treating ingrown hairs. A recent study performed by a dermatologist at the University of Pennsylvania, however, confirmed that treatment with the insulated bulbous probe—a newer type of electrolysis needle sometimes known simply as the *IB probe*—was successful in removing ingrown or very curly hairs.

To find out more about electrolysis and to learn the names of well-qualified, well-trained practitioners in your area, send a stamped, self-addressed envelope to The International Guild of Professional Electrologists, 3209 Premier Drive, Suite 124, Plano, TX 75075.

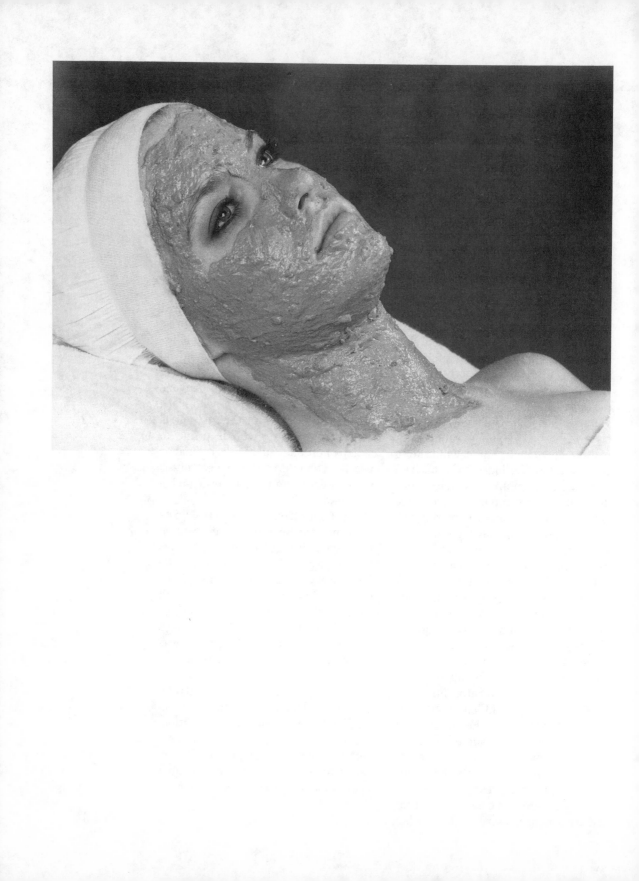

9

Stress
and the Skin

It's no secret that we live in a stressful world today. Whether or not we live in a big city, the pressure to succeed, to make the most of our lives, is all around us. And many women are occupied not only with career goals but with concerns about their families, marriages, and communities. The demands upon our time are great—and sometimes we feel as if we can't do all we'd like. These emotional pressures are translated by our bodies into hormonal stresses, which in turn affect the look and feel of our skin. While stress doesn't really cause skin problems alone, it does aggravate the tendency to have specific complexion concerns. Moreover, when a woman is on the run from home to office to a big evening, it's hard to find time to take care of her skin.

THE HORMONE CONNECTION

Our bodies are very efficient machines, sensitive to myriad cues from our brains; stress activates the very primitive "fight or flight" syndrome, causing stepped-up release of body chemicals (called hormones), which allow us to function on "overdrive" when the going gets rough. Unfortunately, all of this hormone production can upset the skin's oil-to-water balance, with resulting conditions ranging from acne breakouts to exaggerated dryness to serious problems such as eczema and psoriasis.

Stress, however, is a very individual condition. Situations that cause some people to become nervous or fretful, to have trouble sleeping, to overeat, or to skip meals altogether, actually cause other people to thrive on the thrill of a challenge. The first key to managing stress is to evaluate what type of situations put you under pressure and try to manage those events more easily. Many women find that a regular exercise program acts as a wonderful safety valve for the release of stress. Relaxation exercises, yoga, and stretching routines are all good stress relievers, as is going for regular massages or even facials. Remember, too, that stress is as permanent or temporary as *you* choose to make it, and that we, as human beings, can dispel tension if we simply put our minds to it.

Women especially need to learn to take time out for themselves to do what they want to do, even if it's nothing. When you're on the go all day long, simply taking a few minutes of quiet time to read, sew, or leaf through a magazine is important to your well-being. Walking, swimming, or simply spending a few minutes in a sauna or whirlpool can also help to defuse pent-up energy. Scalp treatments and pedicures that include massages of the scalp or feet are also good therapies for our modern stressful world.

WHAT'S YOUR STRESS PROFILE?

Psychologists, who note that none of us would thrive in a world rid of all stresses, a world in which there were never any changes, challenges, or sources of excitement, have devised a system of identifying the events that are the most common—and often unavoidable—sources of stress. These are events that, unlike the short-lived aggravation of having missed your commuter train, do not dissipate within an hour or so, but continue to wreak havoc over time. Many experts agree that if you've experienced several of the events listed below within the past six months or so, you have been under a substantial amount of pressure and are at high risk for a stress-related illness or accidental injury now or in the near future. If you have experienced one of the events on this list, remember that your *reaction* to the stress will help to determine the effect that it has on your mood and your health:

- Has your spouse or partner died?
- Have you become divorced or separated from your spouse?
- Have you separated from your spouse and subsequently been reunited?
- Has a close relative died?
- Have you been hospitalized?
- Have you become pregnant? (Even if you've been aiming to accomplish this for months, pregnancy triggers definite stress.)
- Are you having troubles in your sexual relationship?
- Has your financial situation changed radically—for better or worse?
- Have you or your spouse been fired or laid-off from your job?
- Have you changed jobs?
- Have you had an important job-related success?
- Have you been traveling a good deal and experiencing jet lag on a frequent basis?
- Have you moved to a new city or even to a new home in another area of town?

If you answered yes to at least one of these questions, you are probably under stress. Don't despair. Stress does not mean it's all downhill from here. Being under stress just makes it all the more important to *learn to*

relax. While there is no magic cure for stress, there are proven ways to "defuse" its effects—and even to learn, in some cases, to use stress to your advantage.

RELAXATION
Mind Over Matter

How often have you said to yourself, "Right now, begin to relax"? If you haven't, then you don't know the first key to coping with the unexpected stresses of life. The most successful women are often those who have learned to turn on their relaxation responses whenever times get stressful. What's needed is a realization that when it comes to a woman's emotional and physical well-being, what she doesn't do is as important as what she does. The time spent relaxing, doing nothing, is as important as time devoted to other activities. The more that researchers discover about the essentials of a healthy and long life, the more importance they give to rest and relaxation. Studies at Harvard University, in fact, have revealed that heart-attack patients are helped enormously in their recovery and avoidance of repeated attacks by learning simple relaxation skills. Some of the important attitude changes experts now emphasize:

Learn to say no. One common cause of stress "overload" is taking on too much for the time and resources available. There is a limit to everyone's capacity: Juggling a family, a marriage, a career, and community commitments too often makes us forget our limits. Rather than being angry with you, people around you will usually appreciate your needs—and your honesty—if you let them know you simply cannot take on another commitment. Also, by avoiding taking on more than you can handle, you will find that you do a better job at whatever tasks you do accept, whether they involve time spent with your children, your husband, or your hobby.

Try to balance work with play. It may sound old-fashioned, but it's true. Try to schedule time out with family, friends, or in pursuing a hobby; by scheduling this time, you won't forego it as easily. Also important: Remember that this kind of scheduled relaxation is as vital to your health as any other item on your personal agenda.

Get enough sleep. None of us can stay in top form if we don't get a certain amount of sleep every night. While the exact number of hours varies from person to person, we all know how much we need by the time we are adults. Feeling tired, unenthusiastic, and in need of a nap are all cues that your body hasn't had enough time to "refuel." (You'd be surprised at how many famous, productive people, from Cleopatra to Winston Churchill, relied on daily catnaps.) Try to allow time for a quick rest between your daytime activities and dinnertime; you'll be amazed at the difference that even a few minutes of shut-eye can make.

Learn the art of loafing. Busy women often feel guilty if they spend time doing "nothing." But if you think of an afternoon spent reading, knitting, or simply sitting around and playing games with your children as vital "refueling" time, you'll see that this time is not wasted at all.

Make time for exercise. For many women, exercise is the only time they truly have to themselves, to stop thinking about the worries of the day and simply focus on the pleasure of activity. While we think of exercise as strenuous, one of its most pleasurable results is a feeling of relaxation—probably because challenging our bodies is a great way of work off the steam that often results from a stressful life. Many women who take up a regular exercise routine report that they have less trouble falling asleep and wake up feeling more refreshed than they did when they lived more sedentary lives.

THE STRESS EFFECT
Your Skin's Signals

How to know if your skin troubles are linked to stress? If your skin suddenly becomes oily, develops pimples "under" the skin, or suddenly appears dry, flaky, or itchy, take a few minutes to reflect calmly on the current course of your life. Have you recently taken on a new job or more responsibility in your current job? Are you engaged to be married? Have you suffered a loss of a close friend or family member? Are you moving to a strange city? Both good and bad events can be the source of stress, as any unexpected or major change in the course of your life can lead to all sorts of inner turmoil.

The treatment for stress-induced skin problems is two-fold. First, you should understand the source of your stress and try to do something about it; while we can't eliminate stress from our lives, we can change our approaches and reactions to problems. Trying to look on the bright side of a situation can help to control the oversupply of certain problem-causing hormones in our bodies. Second, and equally important, take steps to help your skin heal itself. If your skin suddenly takes a turn for the worse, it is a good idea to consult a skin care professional, as certain steps that you may think will help your skin to improve could end up worsening a problem. Under stress, most of us develop sensitive skin, along with oiliness or dryness, so we need to be sure that the products we use—cleansers, astringents or toners, and masks—are especially mild. A facial can improve your skin in two important ways. First, by taking time to focus on nothing but yourself, you immediately relax; second, the gentle cleansing and deep-conditioning of your skin will have a lasting impact on its appearance.

I can always tell when clients of mine are under increased stress; their skin not only develops surface problems but also seems to lose the glow that comes from beneath the skin's surface. A woman whose skin is looking less bright than usual might want to use a bit more blusher and apply a brighter-colored lipstick to help create the look of a healthier complexion. If you tend to "take out" tension on your eyes—if they become tired-looking by the end of the day—take fifteen minutes to close your eyes and apply cold cotton compresses soaked in a mixture of equal parts water and milk. The effect will be immediately noticeable.

Finally, remember that all stresses eventually pass—and, often, look a lot less severe in retrospect. Taking a "long" view of life can help to lessen the severity of stress and to improve the look of your complexion—and can also help to decrease facial wrinkles, which are often aggravated if you wear an almost constant frown or walk around with a perpetually furrowed forehead. As my mom used to

tell me when I was young: "If you walk around with that expression on your face, one time it will get stuck that way."

STRESS DEFUSER
A Minisalon at Home

In our busy lives, it is often difficult to schedule visits to a skin care salon at the time that they can do the most benefit: when we are so busy that the reality of spending a half-hour in a softly lighted room having a treatment focused on our appearance and well-being would do wonders for our psyche as well as our skin. The next best thing at that point is to create the ambience and benefits of a relaxing trip to a skin care salon at home. The only essentials are a quiet room with no distractions, with the lights turned down to a soft glow, the phone off the hook or the answering machine on—sort of like hanging the Do Not Disturb sign on your personal door. Perhaps you and your spouse or partner will decide to give each other the following treatments, beginning with fifteen minutes each of detensing massage, using a light cream or lotion applied to the skin first, to cut down on skin friction and allow the movements of the massage to flow smoothly. (Avoid heavy massage oils, as these tend to clog pores; a water-based emulsion-type moisturizer is the best choice.)

Your at-home skin refreshment begins with clean skin. Use a creamy cleanser to wipe away makeup, then a cleansing lotion to remove surface oiliness and dirt; follow with several minutes of warm-water splashes.

Steaming your face is the next, extra-gentle step. Boil a small amount of water and add a tablespoon of chamomile tea. Remove the pan of water from the stove. Apply a moisturizer to your face and neck to protect skin and prevent broken capillaries. Cover your head with a clean towel and form a tent over the towel to prevent steam from escaping; keep your face about 10 inches above the water to avoid the steam's being too hot. (*Note:* Steam should feel warm, not too hot; be careful, as you can easily damage or even burn skin if steam is too hot.) Wait five minutes, then follow the steam treatment with one of the following masks appropriate to your skin type:

Avocado Mask (for dry skin)

Peel an avocado, wash it in lemon water (lemon juice diluted in water) to prevent discoloration, then mash by hand. Smooth onto face and neck and leave on for 10 to 15 minutes, closing

your eyes and lying down with your feet up. Remove with warm, not hot, water and follow with moisturizer.

Yeast Mask (for oily skin)

Dissolve enough dried yeast in warm water to make a thick paste. Apply to face; leave on for 15 to 20 minutes. Remove with warm water. Apply moisturizer.

"Johnny Apple Sage" Mask (for combination skin)

Purée a pared and cored apple and mix with 3 tablespoons honey and a small handful of chopped fresh sage (or a generous sprinkling of dried sage). Blend well; apply to face and wait 15 minutes (put your feet up and close your eyes for the full detensing benefit). Rinse face with warm water; apply a light, water-based moisture lotion.

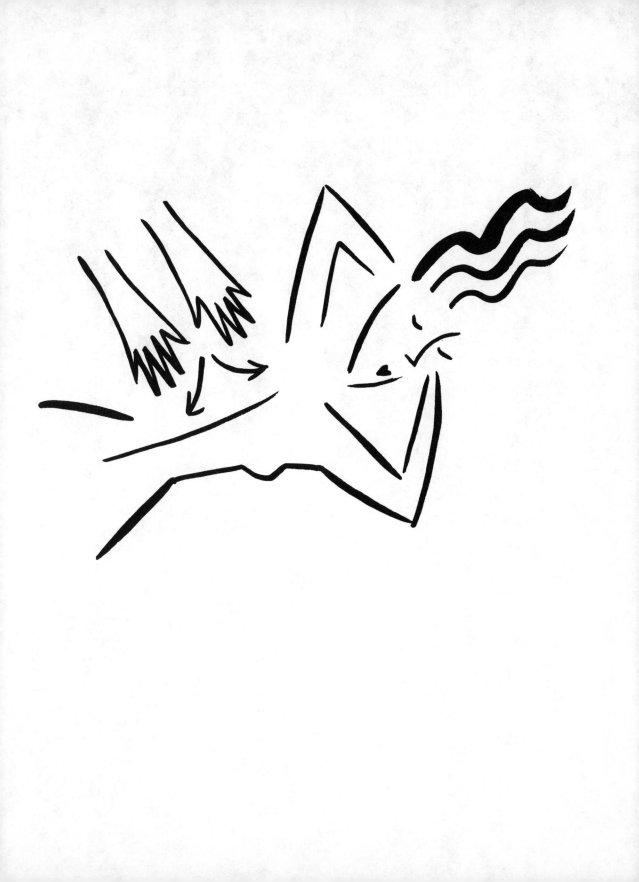

10

Body Care

Most women spend so much time thinking about and caring for their facial skin that they often neglect their body skin. But it's a fact: Skin care does not stop at the neck, but includes the skin from our shoulders down to our toes. In this chapter, I'll show you why paying a little attention to the skin of your body will not only make you look better but feel better as well.

Today, there is new ground being broken in the area of total skin care—in large part, a result of the new attention to health and fitness. It's logical: A woman who spends time on keeping her body in great shape has more reason to care about how the skin of her body looks. She wants her body to be toned and smooth—and she's willing to work at it. The good news is that body care needn't be time-consuming to be effective today. There are not only more options, there are more ways to pamper your skin in less time than ever before.

BODY PERFECT
How Does Your Skin Match Up?

It is always amazing to me how many women who come to my salon cringe at the sight of the slightest imperfection in their facial skin but rarely if ever take note of the appearance of the skin below their shoulders. A facial in my salon includes an examination not only of the skin of the face and neck but a check, too, of the skin of the back and chest—two areas that are especially prone to breakouts in our adult years. Even women who have perfectly clear facial complexions often develop breakouts on the back and shoulders beginning in their twenties or thirties. It is very impor-

tant not to pick at the skin of the back and chest, as it is more prone to scarring than the skin of the face and cannot really be fixed once it is marked.

What causes breakouts on the back and chest? For one thing, the skin of the back and shoulders is thicker and oiler than the skin of the face. Often, breakouts result from oil pooling in these body areas under our clothes, whether due to warm weather outside or stuffiness indoors. As oil collects, it clogs the pores and leads to blemishes. Contrary to myth, blemishes on the back or chest—or anywhere on the body or face—do *not* result from dirtiness and cannot be eliminated through repetitive cleansing. In fact, too-harsh cleansing of the skin in this area often aggravates blemishes and increases the problem.

What to do if you notice blemishes on the back or chest? The best advice is to seek professional cleansing, whether at a skin care salon (be sure that the salon is known for attention to acne) or, if you are unsure of a salon's ability to treat acne breakouts, a dermatologist's office. In either case the treatments will consist of gentle but thorough cleansing using medicated soaps or lotions plus a drying lotion of some type to discourage further breakouts. A "back facial" including a very gentle steaming followed by cleansing may be advised.

The best way to cleanse your back at home is to remove dead cells and impurities while maintaining the skin's natural moisture balance. Hot baths help to dissolve oil and impurities, but if you tend to break out on your back you should really follow a bath with a brisk shower (using hot, then cool, water) to rinse away the dirt and dead cells. I recommend using a cream-formula cleanser in a normal-to-oily skin formula to cleanse the back initially, then following this up with a body scrub that can buff away any patches of dead skin (which can clog pores and lead to blemishes). The back can also be cleaned gently with a loofah or sponge; in most cases, these should not be used on the skin of the chest, which tends to be a little more sensitive. On the chest, I recommend using a gentle lotion cleanser formulated for your skin type, following up with a gentle exfoliating cleanser or scrub product. Don't rub repeatedly with the exfoliating cleanser; instead, gently apply with a circular motion of the fingertips and rinse away with warm or hot water.

If you tend to break out on the back or chest, you may be tempted to use a steam room or sauna to clear up your skin. This is okay if you wash the skin well immediately after leaving the steam room or sauna and apply a drying lotion (such as one containing a camphor base) to any blemishes immediately afterward.

To help prevent perspiration from building up on the body, always wear cotton close to the skin during exercise; not only will it absorb some perspiration but it won't irritate the skin of the body. To prevent clothing from irritating the skin, it's also a good idea to use a gentle rather than harsh laundry detergent, as some detergent residue inevitably builds up within the fibers. (My favorite is Arm & Hammer, as it washes clothes well and leaves fabrics feeling soft and fluffy; its formula is gentle and non-irritating to most skin types.) If you suddenly get a rash on your body after trying out a new detergent, the detergent may be the cause; a dermatologist can determine the culprit.

To give yourself a back facial at home, start with a warm bath. Next, apply a mud-based cleanser; shower off; dry down; then apply a mud-based mask. After fifteen minutes, shower off with warm-to-hot water.

BODY MOISTURE
New Advances, New Pleasure

A few years ago, a woman who wanted to pamper the skin of her body in the same way she did her face had a choice of one or two body lotions, none of which was likely to be formulated any differently from face creams. Today, that has changed; the technology of skin care is now being directed to the specific needs of body skin, which—with the exception of the back and sometimes the chest—is often drier and less smooth than the skin of the face. New, advanced-formula body moisturizers have a double impact on skin, not only leading to a smoother skin surface but working beneath the surface to nourish and hydrate the skin. Apply these lotions immediately after a bath or shower, when skin is still damp. To increase the benefits and the pleasure, apply body creams and lotions with a gentle massage motion. Working with one area of the body at a time, gently smooth a little lotion or cream into the skin; begin massaging with light pressing movements; proceed to a series of kneading movements; and finish with smooth stroking motions. Then, lie down for a few minutes and relax.

THE BATH
Where Body Care Begins . . .

You'll notice that I just said that the best time to apply body creams or lotions is immediately after a bath or shower. Today, skin care experts have learned that the bath can be more than a cleansing routine, that it can actually improve the look and feel of a woman's skin if the proper ingredients are combined. And I'm not talking about old-fashioned bubble baths—I mean a rich, rejuvenating mixture of herbs or oils that will soothe the spirits as well as the skin.

Bathing is not a new beauty idea by any means. As far back as historians can trace, bathing has been recognized as a way to cleanse, relax, nourish, and condition the skin. Beautiful women have had their own personal bathing secrets and recipes. Cleopatra, for example, bathed in milk from horses to keep her skin smooth and soft. Nero's wife, when asked to leave Rome, requested permission to take forty horses with her for this very reason. Nell Gwyn, the mistress of Charles II of England, bathed in rainwater, whereas Chinese queens added oranges to the bath for their invigorating fragrance. Cold bathing was obligatory in Sparta—the idea of "Spartan" beauty treatments is reflected in this tradition! At the Alhambra palace, in Granada, Spain, which was built by the Moors, the bathing areas are among the most beautiful and haunting, with subdued natural light and magnificent tile work.

Today, more and more architects report that increasing attention is being paid to the bathing areas in new houses and apartments. Custom jacuzzis and marble bathrooms are prized features of expensive homes, and we have myriad appliances to make the bath a more luxurious experience. There are high-pressure or massage showers, whirlpool baths, even exercise rooms built into supersize bathrooms. But even if you have

no more than a standard bathtub, you can still make a bath an invigorating, relaxing, rejuvenating beauty experience. Here are some of the best ideas I've culled from my years of experience as a skin care expert:

• To cleanse, cool, and rejuvenate skin in summertime, squeeze the juice of two oranges into a lukewarm bath and soak for ten minutes. Rinse off in a cool shower. Pat skin dry and lavish on a perfumed body lotion.

• To soothe itchy, dry skin, pour 1 cup of vinegar into tepid bathwater. Soak for five minutes. Don't rinse skin; simply apply a rich moisturizing cream immediately after patting skin dry with a soft Turkish towel.

• If you're lacking in energy between the end of the workday and the start of the evening, consider this bath: Add 1 tablespoon of honey to a warm bath. The rich scent and the smoothing effect on your skin will raise your spirits in no time.

• To stimulate your skin and soothe tired muscles after an exercise class, add a cup of buttermilk to a warm bath.

• If you're feeling sluggish, hold a flexible shower head or shower-massage appliance 4 to 6 inches away from your body. Direct a jet of warm water across body skin (not on breasts), moving it back and forth for several minutes. Next, spray a soft zigzag of water up and down your legs. Last, let the water run betweeen inner thighs and calves. Follow up with a cool, invigorating rinse in the shower.

• Beware of routinely adding baking soda to bath water in order to soften hard water. Because baking soda is alkaline (like soap), it attracts natural oils away from the skin and leaves it feeling somewhat dry. Better: bath oil that contains water-softening agents plus oil.

• If your skin feels dry and irritated—especially in the summer, when you've had a little too much sun—add bran, oatmeal, or almond meal to the water (these should be wrapped in a cheesecloth sack to protect the drain).

• Don't take very hot baths. Water that is higher than 95 degrees Fahrenheit can be too drying to your skin, no matter how good it may feel. It's much wiser to stick with 90- to 95-degree water—a temperature that is also just right for dissolving the dirt off of skin. Be especially careful not to take too-hot baths before going out in the evening, as these can sap energy.

• The perfect bath for a weekend athlete who often ends the weekend with sore muscles: Add 1 teaspoon of dried mustard to the bath. It will soothe muscles and relieve stress.

• If you like a fragranced bath, add a few drops of essential oil to the bathwater, or tie a cheesecloth bag filled with fragrant potpourri under the faucet as you let the bathwater run. You may want to avoid fragranced bubble bath solutions as these have been associated with vaginal infections in women who are susceptible to them.

• For ultimate skin lubrication, slather your skin with the highest-grade olive oil before you step into the tub. After a five-minute soak, use a loofah to rub down briskly. (*Note:* Women with sensitive skin should go very easy with the loofah or any other body sponge or washcloth, to protect delicate capillaries from becoming "broken").

• To make an herb bath, fill a mus-lin or cheesecloth bag with herbs and tie it under the faucet as the water flows into the bathtub (or dip the bag into the bath to make an infusion as with a tea bag). For a *stimulating* bath, use basil, bay leaves, fennel, lavender, lemon verbena, mint, rosemary, sage, and thyme; for a *relaxing* bath, use chamomile and jasmine; for a *soothing* bath, use comfrey, marigold, and yarrow; for a *skin-rejuvenating* bath, use blackberry leaves, nettle, and eucalyptus.

• If you are pregnant, do not take very hot baths. Raising your body temperature too high too suddenly can be dangerous (consult your physician about this).

• If you are short on time, consider taking a shower instead of a bath. You can use a scented body scrub, skin-helping mask, or body oil in the shower to make it feel more pampering. Taking a hot shower can feel like a minisauna, relaxing your muscles and giving your body a welcome respite from activity and stress. If you suffer a sunburn, avoid too-hot showers in favor of cool ones. For the best early-morning shower, finish with five minutes of cool rinse at the end; it will get the blood flowing and your energy going.

• For rough, dry patches of skin on elbows, knees, and feet, apply a sloughing mask before a bath or shower. Mix ½ cup sugar and ¾ cup sesame oil, apply to dry body areas, and wait ten minutes. Then slowly rub off the hardened mask with your fingertips, using a circular motion. Follow with a warm shower or bath.

• While running ice cubes over a steaming body may seem like a crazy idea, it's a healthful way to ease into the wonderful sensation of Scandinavian sweat-and-chill bathing—the tradition of going directly from the sauna to the snow that is incredibly exhilarating. How to do it: Tuck a handful of ice cubes into a square of cheesecloth and tie the ends together to make a small bag. Run the bag over your entire body after a hot shower or bath. Towel off; apply fragranced body lotion.

• Exfoliation is the secret of a smooth body complexion. In the shower, use a loofah or a sea sponge. Rub the loofah over your body using long, firm strokes. Follow the bath or shower with a generous application of a rich moisturizer or cream.

• To relax tight muscles, try these three quick exercises in the shower. *Side stretch:* With shoulders relaxed, tilt your head so that your right ear touches your right shoulder. Wait two seconds, then repeat on other side. *Over-the-shoulder stretches:* Turn your head slowly to the left and look over your left shoulder. Wait one second; repeat to other side. *Jaw stretch:* Let your head drop forward, until your chin touches your chest. Hold for a few seconds without tensing your muscles. Now lift your head and let it fall back. Slowly let your jaw drop open and relax. Repeat. (Always use a nonslip mat under you when doing these exercises.)

MASSAGE
The Pleasure Principle

Nothing is more relaxing, invigorating, and therapeutic for the body (and soul) than a massage. It's no wonder that the best skin care salons today offer massage treatments given by trained massage therapists who can isolate your body tension points and help soothe away tight muscles. In addition, properly done professional massage can help increase blood flow and circulation and can be a great way to soothe muscle tightness and soreness after a workout or exercise class. But remember to check ahead of time that the person who gives you a massage has been professionally trained to do the job.

If you've never had a professional massage, the prospect of having one may elicit anticipation and trepidation—after all, massage has a sensual side that can seem a bit off-putting when you're dealing with a total stranger. But keep in mind that a massage is a professional body treatment, although it can also be a wonderful treat between a couple when done at home in private. Because massage is such a private treatment, many women feel most comfortable having their first professional massage done in a skin care salon, by a woman. You should be shown to a dressing room where you change into a robe and slippers and store your clothes, then into the massage room; in smaller salons, your massage room may double as a private dressing room. If heavy oils are used, you may have the option of taking a shower afterward; at some salons, the lightest of body oils are used and the moisturizing ingredients soak into the skin so instantly that a postmassage shower is unnecessary.

The key to getting the full relaxation benefits of a massage is to try to relax completely. Close your eyes and imagine sinking into the table. In some salons, soft music is played during massage treatments to enhance relaxation; often, the lights are dimmed. If certain parts of your body tend to carry tension, tell the masseuse so she can concentrate on those muscles and enhance the massage's benefits.

What makes a professional massage professional is that, while clothes are removed, only the area of the body being massaged at that moment is exposed. The rest of the body is kept covered by a sheet or large bath towel which, besides assuring your privacy, keeps you warm and helps encourage muscles to relax. Different therapists use different types of products to soothe your skin and enhance relaxation. Lotions or oils or even baby powder may be applied to skin to decrease friction; an after-massage rubdown with an alcohol-based toner may substitute for a postmassage shower and help to invigorate your skin and get you moving again.

Most massage therapists use a mixture of different techniques. The two most common types of massage are Swedish (gentle, smooth, gliding strokes and tapping strokes with the heel of the hand) and Shiatsu (a more vigorous massage, derived from Japanese and Chinese techniques, which involves deeper stroking, vibrating, shaking, and cupping movements and is often done with clothing on). Inquire as to the type of massage before making your appointment; some women find Shiatsu a bit rough and not relaxing at all.

If you want to give a friend or lover a massage at home, follow these simple, relaxing steps:

1. Have the person who is receiving the massage stretch out on a comfortable, hard surface (chances are you won't have a professional massage table, so try laying a few blankets on the floor). *Note:* Don't give this massage to a woman who is pregnant or to anyone with a back problem or high blood pressure.

2. Smooth oil or moisturizer on your hands and slide your fingers over one foot. Lightly play with the sole of the foot. Apply more pressure with your thumbs at the points where you feel tension, or little knots.

3. Knead your way up the back of the leg, using your palms and alternating with the balls of your thumbs on the calf muscles.

4. Next, move your hands up the thighs to the lower back. To relax the muscles in the back, knead the muscles of the upper buttocks by lifting the flesh and squeezing it lightly between your thumb and other fingers. Massage the other foot and leg.

5. At the lower back, apply pressure by placing one palm on top of the other. If your hands are starting to meet resistance from the skin, add more oil or moisture lotion. Warm up the back muscles by kneading with the heel of your hands.

6. Run the tips of your fingers gently but firmly up the vertebrae. Working up to the shoulders, concentrate on any areas where you feel tension—usually manifested by hard spots under the skin that are not muscle strength but muscle tightness!

7. Work on any spots of tension by rubbing the balls of your thumbs in a gentle circular motion. Once you've finished, give the person time to relax. Many people actually fall asleep after having a massage, which makes it a perfect bedtime treat.

While a massage seems like a very simple treatment, there are certain times when it is unwise to have one. For instance, a massage should be avoided when you have a fever or infection (massage raises body temperature, which could be dangerous if yours is already high). Anyone who is pregnant or has varicose veins or high blood pressure should also not have a massage. Unless a massage is done by a physical therapist, avoid it if you have an exercise injury. And, though a massage seems like a simple pleasure, be careful not to be over-zealous in giving someone else one: Too much kneading or rubbing can actually induce muscles to tighten up rather than relax. If you're going for a professional massage, remember to look for a *professional*. While, unfortunately, some states do not have legal requirements for massage therapists, many do require licensing. If the state you live in has licensing laws, by all means seek out a licensed practitioner; if not, ask where the therapist received his or her training and whether he or she completed five hundred to a thousand hours of study. If someone balks at answering these questions, stay away; the person probably doesn't have proper credentials. Once you're sure of the therapist's credentials, relax and enjoy: A massage can be the perfect lift to your body and your mind.

BEAUTIFUL BREAST SKIN

The skin of the breasts is thin and delicate and—except in the décolletage area where oil glands are concentrated—natural moisture is scarce and skin is prone to dryness. While skin care should naturally extend to the breasts, many women feel uncomfortable or nervous about treating the skin of this area. There are many myths about breasts in our culture, including the most glaring one promulgated by advertisers that there are exercises or machinery that can increase the size of a woman's breasts.

What is true is that the size of your breasts is a function of genetics, body structure, and body weight. Bust-developing gadgets, massage therapy, or miracle creams simply don't affect the size or shape of your breasts. Even exercise won't dramatically change breast shape, as a woman's breasts don't contain muscles; they're about 80 percent glandular tissue and 20 percent fat.

The one area in which you can change the appearance of your breasts is in the look of the skin. You should cleanse the skin of your body, including your breasts, with a rich emollient soap or shower gel, gently sloughing away any particularly flaky or dry skin with a loofah or sisal mitt. After the shower, while skin is still damp, slather on a rich moisturizing lotion especially suited for body and breast skin. Massage the lotion into the skin gently, working in a circular motion around breasts, then in light, upward strokes. Since the décolletage area is prone to oiliness, apply an oil-absorbing clay- or mud-based mask to this area once a week to prevent blemishes; rinse the mask off in the shower. Because nipple skin is the most sensitive skin of the breast, treat it with extra care. If you don't wear a bra, coat nipples with a dab of Vaseline petroleum jelly to prevent chafing, which comes from friction and perspiration. If nipples do become dry or chapped, soften them with a gentle body lotion.

If you're tempted to bare your breasts to the sun for a truly allover tan, be aware that breast skin is susceptible to burning, and that sun damage can break down elastin and contribute to premature breast sagging. Always protect breast skin with a sunscreen that has an SPF of 10 or above; if this is the first time you are exposing your breasts to the sun, opt for an SPF 15 and cover your breasts after about ten minutes, gradually increasing the sun exposure time over the course of the summer (you will always want to bring a bathing suit top or T-shirt with you to the beach, as a sunburn on your breasts can be especially uncomfortable).

Another time that breasts deserve extra care is during nursing, when it is not uncommon for nipples to feel a bit chafed or raw. To soothe overworked skin, wash with a gentle cream cleanser before and after feedings, ending with a bit of unscented, alcohol-free moisturizing cream.

While many women believe that hair around the nipples cannot be removed, this is not true at all, but is an esthetic judgment. If you want to remove hair from the breasts, you can tweeze the hair in the direction it grows, following up with a dab of alcohol, or opt for the permanent solution of electrolysis (always consult a professional for this last hair-removal option).

Stretch marks on the breast often are the result of pregnancy or a large weight loss. They can also be a simple consequence of the passage of time, a reflection of skin's thinning with age. Nothing can prevent them or take them away once they're there—and they are usually much more noticeable to the woman herself than to anyone who sees her in the nude. Occasionally, stretch marks fade with time if the weight loss occurred during a woman's younger years.

If you want to massage the skin of your breasts, I recommend applying a light massage oil first. Mix 5 drops of lavender oil with 10 drops of juniper oil, 5 drops of rosemary oil, and 5 drops of ylang ylang oil (all are available in health food or apothecary shops). Apply a few drops to the palms of the hands before you begin your massage.

Perhaps the most important benefit of paying attention to the skin care needs of your breasts is that you will become familiar with their normal contour and will have more of a chance of recognizing any change in the shape or feel of your breasts should it occur. Breast self-exams are an essential part of every adult woman's health care routine: if you don't know how to perform a monthly breast self-exam, contact your local chapter of the American Cancer Society to find out, or ask your physician.

THE SPA EXPERIENCE
Total Beauty and Body Care

For the many women who have had the opportunity to spend a few days at a spa, the trip has been a combination of the best of all worlds: time to spend on oneself, time to focus on beauty and health, and time to relax and refocus in an often too-busy life. Today, the possibilities for spa visits are almost endless, ranging from a fast but rejuvenating weekend to an extended, habits-changing stay.

The way to choose a spa is to find out all you can about the facilities and regimen that are offered. At some spas, your day is carefully scheduled, from breakfast to morning exercise classes to lunch and afternoon hikes and massage to dinner and postdinner lectures. Other places focus on doing whatever you please, with a wealth of offerings, including tennis, golf, and water calisthenics, to choose from, but none mandatory. Some spas cater to both women and men, whereas others are for women only; some accommodate hundreds of guests, others a mere thirty per week. At some spas, a range of eating plans, from lavish to Spartan, are offered. At all of the best spas, however, *Spartan* is interpreted in terms of calories; the food you are eating will look as wonderfully appealing and deceptively calorie-laden as the best French restaurant fare. A key question to ask before you go to any spa is the staff-to-guest ratio; pampering comes from almost one-to-one attention, and although it may cost more, many spa-goers feel a stay at a small spa with a large staff is the most wonderful health and beauty investment of all.

Spas in the United States vary from the rigorous Ashram in Calabasas, California, to the luxurious Elizabeth Arden spa, Maine Chance, in Phoenix, Arizona. There are urban spas, such as The Phoenix in Houston or The Greenhouse in Arlington, Texas; or the luxury-retreat spas, such as California's famed Golden Door, or Northern Pines in the forestof rustic Raymond, Maine. What you choose depends on what you're after—a combination spa and family vacation at The Greenbrier in West Virginia, where the spa is truly only an adjunct to the appeal of this wonderful vacation resort, or a true body and mind refocus, such as can be achieved at Rancho La Puerta in Tecate, California.

In Europe, a spa stay is likely to have a slightly different slant than in America. The great European spas are often centuries old and built around a famed natural spring known for its legendary effect on the health of those who drank from it. Those who stay at these spas include Europeans whose physicians have prescribed specific programs as well as more and more Americans seeking exposure to this very different sort of spa life. The exercise programs at European spas are not as varied as in the United States, and the emphasis is more likely to be on improving posture and carriage rather than on building aerobic fitness. Don't expect to find high-tech exercise-monitoring equipment, either. What you will find is a tradition of "taking the waters" and the chance to luxuriate in surroundings that are just what many of us who lead high-stress lives need.

IN THE UNITED STATES

Here is a list of where to go to find more information on some of the best spas around the world:

The Bonaventure
Intercontinental Hotel and Spa
250 Racquet Club Road
Fort Lauderdale, FL   33326
(305) 474-3300

Canyon Ranch
8600 E. Rockcliff Road
Tucson, AZ   85715
(602) 749-9000

Elizabeth Arden's Maine Chance
5830 East Jean Avenue
Phoenix, AZ   85018
(602) 947-6365

The Golden Door
Escondido, CA   92025
(714) 744-5777

The Greenhouse
P.O. Box 1144
Arlington, TX   76010
(817) 640-4000

La Costa Resort Hotel and Spa
Costa Del Mar Road
Carlsbad, CA   92008
(714) 438-9111

The Oaks
Ojai, CA 93023
(805) 646-5573

The Spa At Palm-Aire
2501 Palm-Aire Drive
Pompano Beach, FL 33060
(800) 327-4960

The Palms
572 North Indian Lane
Palm Springs, CA 92262
(619) 325-1111

The Phoenix
111 North Post Oak Lane
Houston, TX 77024
(713) 680-1601

Rancho la Puerta
Tecate, CA 92080
(619) 478-5341

Sonoma Mission Inn
Boyes Hot Springs, CA 95416
(707) 996-1041

In Europe

Biotherm Deauville
Boulevard de la Mer
14800 Deauville, France
(tel.) 98-48-11

Grand Hôtel Beau Rivage
Hoheweg 211
2800 Interlaken, Switzerland
(tel.) 36-21-62-72

Grand Hotel de la Pace
3 via della Torretta
51016 Montecatini
Pistoria, Italy
(tel.) 758-01

Hotel Bristol
3954 Leukerbad
Vallis, Switzerland
(tel.) 27-61-18-33

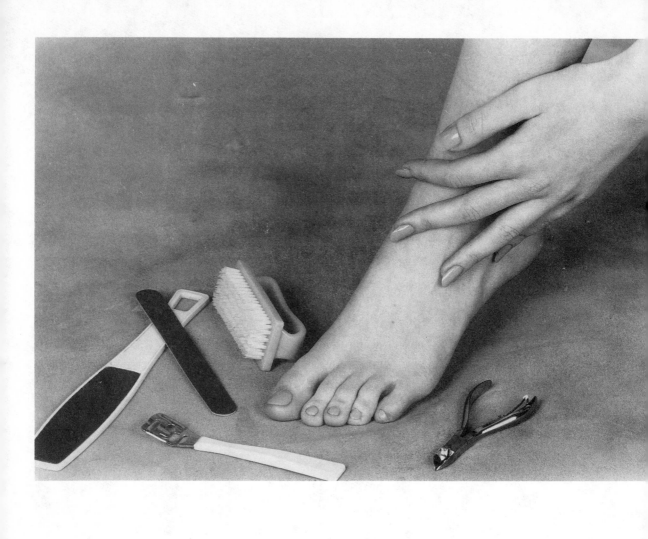

Hands and Feet
The New Beauty
Polish

You may have the best beauty regimen—taking care of your face and body, watching what you eat, and exercising regularly—but don't forget about your hands and feet. Attention to the texture of your skin doesn't stop at the cuff-line of your blouse or trousers: Total skin care is something that shows up in the smoothness of a woman's hands and the attractiveness of well-shaped, highly polished toenails glimpsed through open-toe shoes. A woman's hands and feet carry unspoken messages and reflect attention and pride in appearance. In this chapter, I will share with you my professional advice on manicures, pedicures, and skin protection as well as giving you some time-saving tips for grooming hands and feet.

PROFESSIONAL HANDS
Image-Builders

A woman's hands are not only a symbol of her image, her attention to self-care; they are also hands that work. But today, we don't want our hands to tell the tale of daily labors—we want them to give off a polished image, to look as neat, as professional, as our clothes and our makeup.

This entails paying regular attention to hand care, having regular manicures, and keeping nails trimmed to a "working" length. If there's anything that is a dead give-away of a woman who doesn't take pride in her career, her self, or her job, it is raggedy or broken nails, or nails that are too long or too brightly colored to be taken seriously. That's not to say you have to throw away your bright red nail polish, but to save it for special occasions, or for the weekend.

Getting nail grooming down to a system starts with working out a regular schedule for manicures, which usually means *having a manicure once every two weeks*. Whether you have your nails done professionally or try to maintain them yourself is a matter of personal taste and finances, but it makes the most sense to give your nails at least the head start of being groomed and shaped by a pro once a month, then maintaining them yourself in between visits. If you find you are not able to maintain your nails yourself—as many women aren't—then try to follow my simple, step-by-step instructions for a home manicure in the next section, or, better yet, make a standing appointment with a manicurist at least once every two weeks.

Remember that attractive hands depend on more than good nail condition; the smooth texture and color of your skin also counts. A handshake—a regular part of the business routine—establishes your hands as your calling card; they are the first feature, along with your eyes, that most people notice. Regular hand moisturizing, then, becomes more than a matter of avoiding chapping; it is also vital to keeping hands soft and attractive.

THE PERFECT MANICURE

Giving yourself a manicure at home can be both relaxing and rewarding: Your hands will look better almost immediately, and your nails will stay neat and smooth longer. The manicure I describe here is meant for those times when you can take twenty minutes or a half-hour to give yourself a thorough manicure; when time is of the essence, but you want to improve the look of your hands and nails *fast*, consult the shorter version of this manicure, which I describe in the next section.

1. *Take off old polish.* Soak a cotton ball in an oil-based nail polish remover (never use nail products containing acetone; they make nails dry and brittle) and place it on each nail for twenty seconds to dissolve the polish, then sweep the cotton ball over the nail to remove color. Change the cotton ball as it becomes saturated with polish. Repeat until all polish has been cleansed off of nails.

2. *Smooth your nails' shape.* Use an emery board on the *gentler* side to smooth any rough edges on nails. File in one direction only; do *not* saw back and forth at the nail. Keep the emery board at a 45-degree angle to the nail. To "finish" each nail, stroke the nail lightly up and down with the emery board on the edges. Keep the nail shape straight across at the end, with rounded or squared corners; shaping nails to a narrow end only encourages splitting and breaking of nails. Remember: Take your time to shape and smooth each nail gently; filing with a too-rough emery board or a too-hurried motion can damage nails.

3. *Condition cuticles.* Massage a generous amount of cuticle cream or oil into the cuticle and nail area with your thumb, using circular movements (choose a formula containing nourishing vitamins and natural humectants). Then soak your fingertips for several minutes in a small bowl of warm water, to which you have added a few drops of vegetable, baby, or bath oil.

4. *Moisturize your hands.* Use a soft cotton towel to dry your hands, then massage a rich hand cream into your skin (look for a cream or lotion that contains wheat germ oil, avo-cado oil, and/or peanut oil, all of which are especially nourishing to hand skin). Starting at the end of each finger, gently massage the fingers, one at a time, moving upward toward the wrist. Knead the palm with the fingers of your other hand; switch hands and repeat.

5. *"Squeak" your nails.* Take a small cotton ball and apply a drop or two of nail polish remover to it; quickly run it over your nails to remove any traces of grease to prep the nail for applying polish.

6. *Apply base coat.* If your nails are soft or break easily, this is the time to apply a nail strengthener. Allow it to dry, then apply an acetone-free base coat (as I noted earlier, acetone is a key cause of nail brittleness and damage, so avoid it in all nail care products you use). Allow the base coat to dry.

7. *Apply nail color.* Whatever color you choose, apply it carefully—or all the attention you've paid to shaping and conditioning your nails will be for naught. Start with a line of color going down the center of the nail, then fill in with a line of color on each side. Don't put too much polish on the brush at any one time or you will create ridges in the polish as it dries. Allow the polish to dry thoroughly, then apply a second coat (don't rush this, or you'll end up with bumpy or ridged nail polish). If you want to speed drying along, apply some quick-drying nail spray, available in drugstores or from manicurists, before applying a top coat.

8. *Apply top coat.* Don't skip the clear top coat; these products are formulated to seal in nail color and discourage chipping, which will help maintain your manicure and keep it looking neat for a longer period of time.

9. *Relax your hands.* While you are waiting for the polish to dry thoroughly, take a minute or two to flex and relax your fingers, doing a "dance" on the tabletop. This will help to relax your hands, which can become tense from the concentrated effort of a manicure. Whatever you do, avoid the temptation to rush off to do some chores around the house; touching something before the polish has dried will only lead to smudging and negate all the effort you've put into your manicure.

THE EMERGENCY MANICURE—IN TEN MINUTES FLAT!

There are times when even the most well-groomed woman simply does not have the half-hour it takes to do a complete manicure—times when you look at the clock and realize that you have twenty minutes before your dinner guests arrive, you haven't even begun to get dressed, and your nails are a mess. The good news is that even if you don't have time to do a full, proper manicure, your nails can still look a lot better. The trick: going for an almost nude nail color achieved with—surprise!—ridge filler instead of polish.

First things first: Put on your make-up, get dressed, and take care of any last-minute chores that require using your hands or nails in a manner that could upset your nail polish. Then . . .

1. Strip off your old polish with a nonacetone remover, using a cotton swab to remove any traces of polish that remain under the cuticles.

2. Apply a cuticle cream and gently push back your cuticles with a soft Turkish towel (I'll assume that you've been getting regular mani-

cures, so there's not much need for major "surgery" on your cuticles.)

3. Use the gentle side of an emery board to smooth nails—resist the temptation to reshape your nails, though, as that takes too much time. What you're after is simply smoothing any rough edges that could catch on clothing or make nails look raggedy.

4. Now, take the time to apply a base coat. It takes a relatively short time to dry and will not only help to cover any minor imperfections in nail surfaces but will make your manicure proceed easier and faster. *Don't* use a nail strengthener that contains nail-hardening fibers; these make it more difficult to achieve a smooth finish in a relatively short amount of time.

5. Next, apply a ridge filler, using the following method: With just a little ridge filler on the brush, paint the tip of each fingernail first, then go back and paint the entire nail. The ridge filler will cover the nail smoothly and give you a translucent color midway between pink and white; by painting the tips twice, you'll be covering the part of the nail where the light shows through and where a more concentrated coat of "nude" color is needed. (If you want a bit more color, you could also use the palest pink translucent nail polish, but it will take a little longer to dry and require a little bit more exactitude in application.)

6. Let the ridge filler dry until it isn't tacky. If you're really in a rush, run your hands under icy-cold water to help it set. A method many models use to test the dryness of polish or ridge filler without leaving a mark is touching their tongue *lightly* to the last nail painted.

7. Quickly brush on a topcoat (if you make a mistake or miss a spot

with this, it won't show) and relax until your guests arrive (if time is truly tight, speed the drying time by applying an oil-finish drying coat).

STRONG NAILS
Twenty Tips for an Active Woman

Let's face it. Few of us feel that our nails are perfect and, all too often, they break at the worst possible moment—when we're on the way to a job interview or getting dressed for a formal dinner-dance. While there is no way to guarantee that your nails won't break or peel, there are proven steps that can help to extend the life of a manicure and keep your hands and nails looking their best.

1. *Get a professional manicure every two weeks.* In my opinion, this is really the only way to keep "working" hands looking their best. And putting yourself on a regular bi-weekly schedule allows you to skip a manicure if you're going out of town, or aren't feeling well, or simply don't have the time—without your hands looking rough or your nails ungroomed. Regardless of how handy you are with an emery board or nail polish, I still think that a home manicure is no match for the look that can be achieved by a professional. In between, of course, you'll want to remove your polish and do the abbreviated ten-minute nail-grooming procedure I outlined previously.

2. *Be aware that, while there are no "magic" foods that contribute to nail strength, healthy nails do reflect a healthful life-style.* Despite what our mothers believed, there has never been any solid scientific proof that eating gelatin or any other food makes nails stronger. But eating a balanced diet, exercising regularly, and avoiding health-damaging habits such as smoking cigarettes or over-indulging in alcohol can't hurt nails and may even help. The premise is that because nails are not essential to health, our bodies will naturally scrimp on their strength when other parts of our bodies need more restorative attention.

3. *Protect your hands from the elements.* In winter, don't go outdoors without gloves, even if it's just for a minute; dryness is a key cause of nails, splitting, chipping, and breaking. If you're washing dishes or gardening, the same advice applies.

4. *Apply hand cream constantly.* It is literally impossible to overmoisturize your hands or your cuticles, so keep a tube of hand cream in your desk drawer, inside your attaché case, near the kitchen sink, and on your bedroom vanity table, and apply as often as possible, especially—and immediately—after washing your hands or coming indoors from the cold.

5. *Protect your hands from the sun.* Our hands are one skin area that can give away our ages instantly. Because sun exposure contributes to the formation of brownish age spots, applying sunscreen regularly will help keep hands looking younger longer. In fact, many dermatologists today recommend applying sunscreen to face *and* hands daily, to prevent the cumulative damage of daily sun exposure. For this reason, you might want to choose a sunscreen in a rich moisture base to use instead of hand cream, at least in spring and summertime, when hands are not protected by gloves.

6. *Use a rejuvenating mask on the hands once a week.* The face is not the only skin area that can benefit from a moisturizing mask. Next time

you take the time to apply a mask to your face, treat your hands to one as well. Choose a mask that is rich in moisturizing ingredients such as avocado oil or sesame oil rather than a tightening mask, which is not good for the constantly exposed skin of the hands. You'll be amazed at how much smoother and softer your hands will feel after even one concentrated moisturizing treatment.

7. *Smooth away rough spots with a pumice stone after you take a shower or bath.* Another skin-smoothing tool that we rarely think of using on our hands but that works wonderfully is a pumice stone, or even a loofah sponge. Either of these tools should be used very gently on skin that has been soaked in water first (as in a shower or bath). Use only on rough spots and follow by rinsing in lukewarm water, patting skin almost dry with a towel, and applying a rich lubricating moisturizer.

8. *Give your hands an overnight moisture treatment once a month.* Before going to bed, apply petroleum jelly or a very rich moisturizing cream to hands and put on cotton gloves. As you sleep, the gloves will hold in body heat and help the cream or lotion to penetrate the skin of your hands. In the morning, take off the gloves and use a clean towel to pat off any excess cream. Your hands will feel wonderfully soft and smooth.

9. *Try to avoid using scissors or clippers on fingernails whenever possible.* Metal tools tend to encourage nails to split or to become brittle; stick to the gentle side of emery boards instead.

10. *Don't file nails too close to the sides.* If you can, rely on a professional manicurist to give your nails their basic shape and simply follow that shape in your home touch-ups.

Aim for a gently rounded, not a square or pointed, shape; this is not only the most modern look, it is also the shape that gives your nail length the most natural support.

11. *Always use acetone-free nail polish remover.* While the solvent acetone is the fastest at dissolving nail polish, it also tends to dry out nails and is also a potential skin sensitizer. Using an acetone-free remover may take a few more seconds, but it's worth the extra time in ensuring nail health. A final note of caution: Resist the temptation to peel off nail polish; you're likely to peel off the top layer of your nail along with the polish.

12. *Give your nails a rest from polish in between manicures.* While it is true that nail polish acts as a protective coating on nails, adding to nail hardness and helping to prevent breakage, keeping nails under cover all the time can lead to staining and, sometimes, dryness. It's a good idea to let your nails breathe for a weekend, or even a day or so, in between your biweekly manicures.

13. *Be cautious in the use of nail hardeners.* Products that contain formaldehyde can cause allergic reactions such as rashes as well as irritation. Nail-hardening formulas that are labeled *hypoallergenic* are less likely to cause problems; they usually contain alkyl polyester resins instead, and help to thicken the keratin (outer-most) layer of the nail. Many dermatologists, feel that the best way to decrease nail breakage is to use a nail *conditioning*, not a hardening, product. I agree. The proteins or waxlike lipids in nail conditioners have been shown to form a film over the nail's surface and to keep nails moist and pliable, making them the most resistant to tearing; in some studies proteins such as collagen

were even shown to penetrate the nail plate and become incorporated into the structure of the nail itself.

14. *Buff your nails regularly—but don't overdo it.* Buffing brings up the pinkness and natural sheen in your nails, but overdoing it can actually remove the uppermost layer of nail proteins, weakening the nail structure. As a general rule, experts recommend buffing nails once a week and not more often, and using a buffing cream to act as extra protection between the nail and the buffer. The best method is to buff diagonally across the nail in one single long, firm stroke. Don't buff too vigorously; you can literally burn nails with too much friction. To take advantage of the improvement in nails' natural color and glow after buffing, you might want to buff your nails on the days you choose to take a breather from wearing nail polish.

15. *Be gentle with cuticles.* The biggest source of disagreement among nail care professionals themselves is whether to push back or trim cuticles. Dermatologists, however, note that the less you do to your cuticles, the better the condition of nail growth is likely to be. I prefer pushing back cuticles as gently as possible, always applying a cuticle cream or oil first, then pushing back with a gentle tool such as a Turkish towel wrapped around a fingertip or a cuticle stick wrapped with soft, absorbent cotton. Never trim cuticles unless absolutely necessary; cutting too close can damage the nail bed—the source of future growth—and lead to spotty or pitted nail growth in the future.

16. *Use a white pencil to touch up yellowed nail tips.* The cause of yellowed nail tips includes, of course, smoking cigarettes but it can also in-clude wearing dark-colored nail polish, especially if you've skipped a base coat, or simply working with household cleaners, dyes, or hair colors. White pencil can work as a nail "makeup" when you wear sheer or clear polish, or no polish at all. To use, first moisten the point of the pencil, then apply to the underside of clean nails with a gentle circular motion, and finish with a clear coat of polish applied to the underside of nail as well as the top surface. Don't use the plastic cap on the pencil to clean your nails; it is not pointed enough and is too stiff to be safe. Use a round-edged wooden manicure stick instead.

17. *Get the most out of your nail polish by storing it properly.* Store nail polish in a dry, cool place. Another tip to keep polish fresh longer is to wipe the neck of the bottle after each use, so polish doesn't accumulate there, making it impossible to close it tightly. A bottle of polish that is not closed tightly will become thickened or tacky. If this happens and you don't have the time to buy a new bottle, add a drop or two of nail polish solvent (sold in most drugstores alongside nail colors) to the bottle, close the bottle cap, and shake vigorously to thin polish out to the point at which it will again glide onto nails easily.

18. *Have nails "wrapped" by a professional only.* While nail wrapping can help to support weak nails as they grow longer, when done improperly, it can actually hasten nail breakage close to the quick, risking lasting nail damage. Artificial nail tips should also be applied *only* by professionals, as they can cause problems as well if improperly used. Acrylic nails have been the subject of many complaints from dermatolo-

gists, as they have caused many problems (even, in some cases, nail loss). Always go to a respected salon to have nail tips applied and be sure that the nail extensions used there are not the type that cover the entire nail; these total-coverage artificial nails have been known to suffocate new nail growth underneath. If extensions are used at all, they should be applied only to the tips of your nails and should not be so long that they will catch on clothes and be likely to break.

19. *Consult a doctor if nails become discolored or bend at the tips, or if red, scaly patches develop on the skin of the hands.* Hand and nail problems can go beyond the cosmetic concerns I've dealt with here and be real medical problems. Allergic reactions, rashes, and dermatitis can all develop on the hands as well as the face. If this happens, see a dermatologist, who can diagnose the cause and recommend treatment.

20. *If you are pregnant, enjoy the benefits to your nails.* Many women find that the hormones secreted by the body during pregnancy have a positive effect on the appearance of their nails, speeding growth and adding to strength. Unfortunately, there is often a corresponding increase in nail breakage and weakening after the child is delivered. But, meanwhile, enjoy!

HAND REVIVERS
Fast Finger Play

After a day spent working with your hands—whether around the house, at a typewriter or computer, or writing out wedding invitations—your hands may feel tired, stiff, in need of being energized. A no-fail trick: Hold your hands overhead, inhale deeply, and count to five, then exhale slowly while lowering your hands to your sides. Then, shake both hands vigorously while holding them loosely from the wrists. Repeat both steps several times. As a finishing touch, smooth on a silky hand lotion and massage it into each finger, from the base to the fingertips, and then into the palms of each hand.

When your hands feel fatigued during the day, take a minute out to massage them: Open the palm of one hand and use the opposite fist to massage the inside of the palm in a circular motion; repeat with opposite hand.

THE PERFECT PEDICURE
An Essential Beauty Treatment

Today, most of us spend a good deal of time on our feet—walking to work, exercising, or standing up as part of our jobs. For comfort as well as a neat, clean image, a pedicure is a must; there is nothing very attractive, for example, about a woman who is dressed for a black-tie dinner with rough-skinned heels showing through a pair of sling-back shoes, or unpolished, ungroomed toenails showing through open-toed summer pumps. Every woman who has ever had a professional pedicure will attest to how relaxing it is, as well as how wonderful it feels.

Foot grooming begins with cleanliness, which means cleansing your feet every day just as carefully and gently as you do your face. A woman who exercises should be especially careful to dry and powder between her toes to cut down on perspiration and foot odor. You should allow any exercise shoes to air out between wearings to avoid perspiration buildup, which not only can lead to odor but can also cut down on the life span of your shoes by eating away at the inner supportive lining.

Here is a basic home pedicure to keep your feet looking sleek in and out of sneakers and shoes (ideally, use this pedicure as a treatment in between regular monthly professional pedicures).

1. *Soak feet in warm, soapy water for five to ten minutes.* Add a moisture-rich skin cleansing formula to the water, one that's intended for dry or sensitive skin and that has a fresh, but not too heavy, fragrance.

2. *Smooth rough skin on heels and balls of feet.* With a pumice stone or grainy cleanser, gently rub away rough or scaly skin, concentrating on areas, such as balls of feet or edges of toes, that take the most "shoe abuse."

3. *Trim nails straight across.* If you have a regular pro pedicure, then just use the gentle side of an emery board to smooth away any rough edges on toenails, maintaining the established nail shape. If you're doing your own pedicures on a regular basis, use a toenail clipper to clip nails straight across—being certain not to clip any closer than the ends of your toes, as cutting nails too short is one of the most common causes of ingrown nails. Use an emery board to file away any rough edges gently, but don't saw back and forth.

4. *Push back cuticles gently.* After applying a cuticle lotion or cream, use a towel-wrapped finger to push back cuticles gently; if you feel yours need more help, then wrap several layers of cotton around an orange stick and use that instead. In general, do as lit-

tle manipulating of cuticles as possible, as it is very easy to upset future nail growth by being overzealous with cuticle trimming or pushing. Avoid cutting cuticles unless they are very long and raggedy. Use the towel or cotton-wrapped orange stick to clean under the edges of toenails.

5. *Massage feet.* Using a rich moisturizing lotion (a hand or body cream is fine), gently massage the tops and bottoms of feet as well as individual toes. Try the following relaxation-promoting technique: Grasp one foot with both hands, thumbs on top of feet, and stroke from heel to toe back and forth for a minute or so, until you feel the muscles and ligaments of the foot relax. Take each toe and gently rotate it in a circle. Flex foot back and forth, then use your thumbs to massage the top of the foot from ankle down to toes; repeat the same technique on the underside (sole) of the foot. Repeat the entire massage technique on the other foot.

6. *"Squeak" nails clean.* Using a cotton ball dipped in nonacetone nail polish remover, cleanse away any residue of moisture lotion on toenails.

7. *Prepare toes for nail polish.* Using rolled-up or twisted facial tissues or pedicure pads, separate toes so that they don't touch.

8. *Apply nail polish.* As with a manicure, start with a clear base coat, then two coats of your favorite color polish (the one place where bright, bright nail polish looks very chic is on toenails).

9. *Relax while polish dries, then finish with a clear top coat.* Take a few moments to close your eyes, relax while nail color dries. Then apply a clear top coat and let it dry thoroughly before removing toe-separating tissues or pedicure pads.

SLEEK FEET
Ten Foot-Caring Tips

Just as you take certain important steps to protect the look of your hands, you can also practice what I call "foot smarts" to keep your feet in good condition all year round. Here are some of the most important foot-caring steps:

1. *Apply a moisturizer to your feet every night.* Just as you moisturize your face and hands every night, apply a moisturizing lotion or cream to your feet as well.

2. *Add body oil to your bath to keep skin soft and smooth.* A bath oil will not only help smooth the skin of your body; it will also help to keep your feet moisturized. If you don't want to use a fragranced oil, you can use pure avocado oil instead.

3. *Always wear socks with sneakers or tennis shoes.* The only time you can go sockless without concern is when you're wearing all-leather sandals. Otherwise, perspiration will become trapped against your skin and will add to skin roughness and irritation, and even, in the most severe cases, contribute to the skin irritation known as athlete's foot.

4. *Give your feet an "oatmeal treat."* In the bath or shower, rub uncooked oatmeal mixed with an equal amount of cornstarch onto wet feet; this will gently rub away dead, flaky skin. Rinse well; pat feet dry with a towel; apply moisturizer.

5. *Try this soak for "beat feet."* After you've been on your feet all day, soak them in cool (not hot) salted water for five minutes; rinse with clear, cool water; pat dry with a towel. Then massage your feet with a cooling moisturizing gel or cream. Lie down and elevate your feet above your hips for five minutes to allow the moisturizer to be absorbed by skin.

6. *Wear well-fitting shoes.* Many women add to foot discomfort by choosing shoes that are fashionable but do not fit well; sacrificing fit for fashion is not wise at all. Experts recommend that there should be at least one-sixteenth of an inch between the end of your big toe and the tip of a shoe, and that all straps should "give" slightly, not pinching the foot. In addition, low- to medium-height heels will be more comfortable as the day goes on than very high, thin heels.

7. *Use foot powder if your feet tend to perspire.* A powder that combines talc with cornstarch is best for absorbing perspiration. If in doubt, ask a druggist for a recommendation.

8. *Exercise your feet to relaxation.* When you come home after a long day, try this foot-reviving workout before getting dressed to go out at night: Scatter a few pencils on the floor and pick them up with your toes. Then straighten your toes and rotate your ankles first to the left several times, then to the right. Then fill a pair of moccasin-style slippers with a handful of dried beans, slip your feet inside, and walk around the bedroom several times—you'll get a massage-like workout on the soles of your feet.

9. *Always cut toenails straight across.* Cutting in too close on the sides increases the risk of developing painful ingrown toenails.

10. *Give your feet a thalassotherapy massage at home.* If you've ever visited a spa, especially in Europe, you've probably experienced the wonderful combination of water and massage. Here's a mini-thalassotherapy treat for your feet: Sit on the edge of the bathtub and give your feet a bath under the faucet; alternate one min-

ute of hot water with one minute of cold, ending with cold (if you have a shower massage attachment, use this instead of the faucet). Then get out of the bath and pat feet dry, paying special attention to the areas between the toes. Next, massage moisturizer into feet and up to calves with smooth, even, upward strokes of your fingers and palms. Pull on and gently rotate each toe for a few seconds. Finally, powder feet to preserve the fresh feeling.

ON-TARGET QUESTIONS
Hands and Feet

Q: What can I do to strengthen my very soft nails?

A: Many people believe in using nail hardeners to solve this problem, but they are only a temporary solution, as they work only as long as you keep applying the nail-hardening formula on a regular basis. Another good idea is to soak your nails in warm avocado oil rather than warm water during a manicure. Or seek out a manicurist at a beauty salon who uses warm moisturizing cream instead of warm soapy water for a prepolish soak. To help the nail from where it grows, apply cuticle cream several times a week and always keep at least two coats of polish on nails at all times to act as a barrier to breakage.

Q: I exercise a great deal and have developed rough skin on the soles of my feet due to perspiration. What should I do?

A: Postexercise, soak your feet in warm water in which you have sprinkled a handful of Epsom salts, then use a grainy cleanser to work on any rough skin spots. Follow up with a creamy moisturizer. And always sprinkle powder on your feet before putting on your sports socks and allow your sneakers to air out between wearings.

Q: I have regular manicures but when I grow my nails longer, then tend to snap. What is wrong?

A: Perhaps you are simply growing your nails *too* long. For both practicality and a modern, attractive look, don't grow your nails much longer than half an inch from the end of your fingers; any longer and you will have the look of a woman who doesn't work—because long nails do make it impossible to use your hands for anything more than decoration without your nails breaking.

Q: I recently began a regular running program and find that my feet have developed an unpleasant odor. What should I do?

A: Foot odor from running—or any other regular exercise—can come from the combination of perspiration and the natural buildup of dead skin. In the wet, warm environment of a pair of workout shoes, bacteria have all the conditions they need to thrive, so you should be vigorous in foot cleansing and perspiration control.

Always wash your feet with an antibacterial (in other words, deodorant) soap daily, dry thoroughly, paying special attention to the area between your toes, and use an antiperspirant/antibacterial talcum powder before putting on your socks. If this doesn't help, you may have a more serious foot problem and should consult a dermatologist.

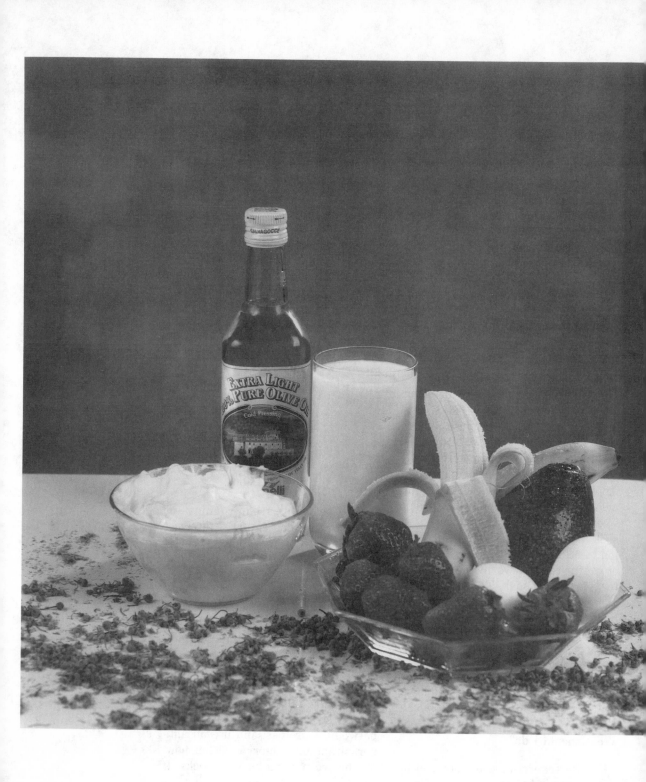

12

Feeding your Skin

A well-balanced diet is essential to proper skin care—it is the inner beauty regimen that complements your daily skin care routine. In many ways, the look of a woman's skin, hair, and nails reflects the state of her inner health; deficiencies and ill health show up almost immediately in a lack of skin color, a change in hair texture, brittleness or breakage of nails. Yet it is also true that in the past few years American women have in many cases been sold a bill of goods when it comes to nutrition, as less than honest companies have tried to convince us that a specific vitamin pill—or herbal drink—holds the one and only solution to perfect skin and health. If you are looking for a magic formula, I suggest you look elsewhere; today even nutrition scientists agree that there is only so much we understand about the connection between diet and health.

WE ARE WHAT WE EAT

Whoever coined that phrase knew what he or she was talking about. Unfortunately, the reality of modern life doesn't allow many of us time to prepare or enjoy a truly balanced diet. When I ask my clients whether they eat a balanced diet the most common response is "Who has the time?"

Yet, contrary to popular thought, it doesn't take a great deal of time to eat healthfully. It is just as easy to stop at a salad bar on your way home from work as it is to stop for a hamburger; the difference between eating fresh vegetables and overcooked hamburgers is not one of time but commitment to a healthful style of eating. One glance at the menus in many of the best restaurants shows you that it is as simple to order plain broiled fish as it is to ask for fish smothered in rich cream sauce; if you have an interest in your long-term health, you'll skip the sauce. Shopping at the supermarket offers nutrition-wise choices even for those who hate to cook; there are frozen dinners that are low in fat and salt in every supermarket in the country.

In short, eating a balanced diet is not difficult; it simply requires making proper choices from the multitude of foods available to us today. Here are several simple steps that will help to put your diet on the right track:

Don't eat the same thing every night. The first step, nutritionists agree, in getting the forty-plus nutrients that our bodies need to maintain health is to eat a variety of foods. While this sounds elementary, I can't tell you how many women I know who now eat the same green salad for lunch and can of water-packed tuna for dinner every day because they are convinced this is the way to lose weight. Even when you're on a weight-loss diet, your body needs a variety of foods to maintain energy and health. The greater the range of foods you eat every day, the less likely you are to develop low-grade deficiencies that can sap energy and health.

The simplest way to put variety in your diet is to make selections from each of the following major food groups daily (figure roughly ½ cup per serving):

1. Fruits and vegetables (four or more servings daily)
2. Cereals, whole-grain and enriched breads, and grains such

as rice, pasta, and bulgur (at least four servings daily)

3. Meats, poultry, eggs, fish *or* dry peas and beans (soybeans, kidney beans, black-eyed peas, lima beans) (two servings daily)
4. Low-fat milk, cheese, or other dairy products (at least four servings daily)

Avoid overeating. Being overweight is not only unattractive; it poses a long-term risk to a woman's health. Obesity increases your chances of developing high blood pressure, diabetes, and heart disease, note studies supported by the U.S. Department of Health, and Human Services.

Some strategies to prevent overeating: Plan what you are going to order before you arrive at a restaurant. When it's your choice, choose a restaurant that offers low-fat options on its menu. Skip high-fat condiments such as creamy salad dressings, butter on your bread, and sour cream or butter on your baked potato. Don't hesitate to order an appetizer as your main course after starting with a mixed salad; even the most expensive restaurants now acknowledge that many of us are trying to eat less than in the past.

Eat more than once a day. If you have discovered that you're not losing weight by skipping lunch, you may actually be sabotaging your efforts. Many people who skip breakfast and/or lunch get so hungry at night that they overeat at dinner, without realizing that food eaten late at night may not be burned off at the same rate that food eaten earlier in the day—when activity is highest—is used up by the body. Eat a bigger lunch and a much smaller dinner and

you may be able to put your weight back in control.

Avoid too much fat and cholesterol. Scientists have proven a correlation between the amount of fat in Americans' diets and our risk of diseases including heart disease. Cutting down on cholesterol doesn't mean you can no longer eat any animal products or meat; it does mean making certain simple choices, such as eating meat less frequently, or skipping the mayonnaise in your tuna salad, or eating fewer desserts topped with whipped cream. Some simple tips for cutting back on the fat in your diet:

1. Choose lean meat, fish, skinned poultry, dry peas, and beans as your protein sources. Be aware that meat is graded by its fat content, with prime steak the highest in fat of all. When preparing meat, trim away all visible fat *before* and *after* cooking.
2. Moderate your intake of eggs and liver.
3. Avoid foods in which butter, cream, or hydrogenated oils are listed as primary ingredients. Look for more healthful safflower, sunflower, soybean, or olive oils.

Eat foods that provide adequate fiber. Eating more fiber will give you a fuller feeling if, like many women, you're trying to eat less and lose a little bit of weight. Allowing your body to cleanse itself naturally without the use of artificial laxatives can also help to balance your skin's self-cleansing process. There is also growing evidence that eating a diet rich in fiber may help to prevent certain types of cancer and adult-onset diabetes.

Where to find fiber: in natural-grain breads and cereals, fresh fruits and vegetables (celery, kiwi, and carrots are prime examples), and, of course, in products such as wheat germ, which can be sprinkled into any type of recipe to increase the fiber content. Cooking decreases the fiber in foods: We eat too many processed or overcooked snacks and dishes. When possible, remember that fresh—as in fresh vegetables, fruits, and whole-meal grains—is better than canned, frozen, or cooked.

Eat more complex carbohydrates. Recent nutrition research shows that complex carbohydrates—found in pasta, potatoes, whole grains, rice, and breads—provide the best fuel for the body. Nutritionists now believe that if more of our diets consisted of complex carbohydrates, our society would have lower rates of many types of disease. And, contrary to what many women were brought up to believe, complex carbohydrates are not fattening (too often, it's the buttery or creamy sauces and toppings we add to them that are, so you'll want to switch your preparation).

Avoid too much sugar and salt. Studies show that the average American consumes as much as 130 pounds of sugar in a year! Sugar, honey, jams, and jellies are primarily empty calories, providing a quick burst of energy that disappears as quickly as it comes, giving the body no fuel to draw upon as the day goes on.

Besides skipping the sugar when you take your morning cup of coffee and bowl of breakfast cereal, there are other ways to cut down on the sugar in your diet. Have a pumpernickel or whole-grain roll at your coffee break, not a Danish. Learn to appreciate the natural sweetness of fresh orange slices for dessert rather

than cookies, candies, or canned fruit. And be aware that *sugar* is usually not listed as an ingredient in prepared foods, although they are sweetened; the ingredients sucrose, glucose, maltose, dextrose, or fructose all indicate sugar has been added to a food's preparation.

It is also smart to cut down on salt. Learn to taste your foods before you season them; you may be surprised at how wonderful they already are without added salt. Also, watch out for salt added to canned vegetables or soups, as well as to stuffing mixes or prepared pasta dishes. Of course, staying away from salted snack foods such as pretzels or corn chips makes sense, as does reading labels of products such as antacids—often incredibly high in sodium. Aside from multiplying a woman's risk of developing high blood pressure—a health problem affecting roughly 17 percent of adults in this country—salt has another undesirable side effect. A high salt intake is a key cause of water retention, giving your body and your face a bloated appearance. Proof positive: One woman who comes to my salon who recently went on a low-sodium diet to decrease her blood pressure suddenly noticed that the bags under her eyes seemed to disappear in a matter of weeks; unbeknown to her, the water she was retaining in her body was also being deposited in her face!

VITAMINS AND MINERALS
Magic Nutrients?

Despite what you may read on the vitamin bottle, vitamins alone cannot provide your body with instant energy or instant health. Vitamins are essential to your body's proper functioning but they don't work alone—in fact, vitamins' action within the body is limited to converting *food* into useful energy. While vitamin deficiencies are certainly dangerous, doctors today are seeing increasing cases of patients who are suffering from vitamin *over*doses, caused by taking too many vitamins in the mistaken belief that if one vitamin pill is good for you, then more will be even better. The average woman who eats a healthful diet does not need anything more than a basic once-a-day multivitamin and mineral supplement, say nutritionists. If you feel you need to take more than that, check with your doctor.

To put together the following guide to vitamins and minerals, I went to nutrition experts from the U.S. Department of Agriculture. Here is what these experts have to say:

All vitamins fall into two basic groups, water- or fat-soluble. *Water-soluble vitamins* are literally those that dissolve in water; if these vitamins are not used up by the body, they are excreted in urine and sweat. *Fat-soluble vitamins*, on the other hand, are stored within the body's fat cells, which means that if you take too much of a fat-soluble vitamin, it will stay within the body, where, in some cases, it can build up to dangerous levels. The eight B vitamins and vitamin C are water-soluble; the huge amounts of these vitamins that are taken by many Americans are often quite literally washed down the drain. The fat-soluble vitamins A, D, E, and K don't need to be replenished to any degree beyond the amounts normally found in a well-balanced diet.

Minerals, while stored in the body, can be depleted by physical and emotional stress. The minerals present in the largest quantities are calcium, chlorine, magnesium, phosphorus,

potassium, sodium, and sulfur. Experts feel that American women get all they need of these macrominerals with the important exception of calcium. So-called trace minerals (aluminum, cadmium, copper, fluoride, iodine, and lead) are found in the body in tiny but crucial amounts; we do not need to supplement these minerals.

Here is a quick summary of the role that the major vitamins and minerals play in the body, plus foods that are good sources of each.

Fat-Soluble Vitamins. Experts recommend that these vitamins not be supplemented except under a doctor's close supervision:

Vitamin A is important in the growth and repair of tissues. Adequate vitamin A intake helps to keep the skin smooth and infection-free. A deficiency of vitamin A can show up in exceedingly rough, dry skin; ridged or peeling fingernails; or even blackheads, in some cases. Good sources for vitamin A in your diet are eggs; yellow, orange, or dark green vegetables (such as carrots, spinach, and broccoli); and liver. (*Note:* Overdoing your intake of vitamin A-rich vegetables can give your skin a yellowish orange tinge. Although not dangerous in itself, this can be an important warning sign if you keep eating these vegetables at the same rate, you can develop vitamin A toxicity.)

Vitamin D aids in the formation and maintenance of healthy teeth and bones by helping the body to absorb calcium and phosphorus. Look for vitamin D in milk, egg yolks, liver, tuna fish, and salmon.

Vitamin E plays a role in the cells'

ability to utilize oxygen as well as helping in general circulation. Good sources of Vitamin E are foods such as cold-pressed vegetable oils (wheat germ oil, corn oil, margarine) and raw seeds and nuts, as well as green, leafy vegetables and whole-grain cereals.

Vitamin K helps blood to clot. A deficiency of this vitamin is extremely rare, as it is needed in very, very small amounts and is found in a wide variety of foods ranging from green, leafy vegetables to cabbage, cauliflower, and potatoes to cereals, yogurt, and egg yolks.

Water-Soluble Vitamins. While not readily stored by the body, water-soluble vitamins are very easily available within a balanced diet and need not be taken in high doses.

B-complex vitamins have been called the "stress vitamins" by some experts, because they are thought to be depleted by physical and emotional stress. Deficiencies can cause dry, cracking skin, especially around the edges of the lips and nose. Good sources of the B vitamins are brewer's yeast, liver, whole-grain cereals, pork, peanuts, and leafy green vegetables.

Vitamin C, while it does assist the body in the healing process, has never been scientifically proven to have any influence on whether or not you catch a cold or how long the cold lasts. Drinking a single glass of orange juice each morning actually gives your body all the vitamin C you need every day! Other good sources are citrus fruits, tomatoes, strawberries, melons, potatoes, and green peppers and other dark green vegetables.

Minerals. Here is a rundown of the most common minerals required in a woman's diet:

Calcium, as anyone who reads the popular press well knows by now, is an essential mineral and one that far too many women don't get enough of. Aside from being essential to healthy teeth, calcium can help to prevent the bone-thinning disease known as osteoporosis. What many women don't realize is that getting adequate calcium in your diet can also help to keep your skin smooth and aid in your complexion's natural self-healing processes. Good sources of calcium include milk (choose low-fat or skim), cheese, egg yolks, beans, lentils, nuts, figs, cabbage, cauliflower, and asparagus.

Iodine, which is essential to proper functioning of the thyroid gland, has been implicated in causing acne eruptions in adulthood by some dermatologists. Some women, they think, are especially vulnerable to excess iodine intake, and this vulnerability shows up in skin reactions. The fact is, experts note, that because our salt intake is so high and most of the salt used is iodized (has iodine added to it), many of us unknowingly get much more iodine in our diets than is necessary for health. Doctors recommend that women who develop acne breakouts in adulthood try to cut down on their intake of salty foods, seafood, and products containing seaweed, and see whether the results include a clearing of skin problems.

Iron is important to the production of hemoglobin, which is an essential blood constituent that helps to maintain energy level, skin color, and nail strength. Good sources of iron include leafy green vegetables, liver, and oysters. While many nutritionists feel that most American women—and especially those who are especially active—may need iron supplements in order to meet their daily recommended intake, they urge women to consult a professional before supplementing this mineral.

Magnesium helps to prevent tooth decay and aids in proper functioning of the nerves, including those that carry messages to the skin surface. Good sources include fresh green vegetables, nuts, soybeans, and peas.

Phosphorus is involved in aiding just about every body function, most importantly the growth and repair of cells and prevention of fatigue. Excessive intake of carbonated beverages has been implicated by some experts in upsetting the body's phosphorus balance. Good sources include meat, fish, fowl, eggs, nuts, and whole grains.

Potassium helps to regulate the body's fluid balance in conjunction with sodium and is important to normal growth, healthy skin, and general metabolism. While some exercise teachers tout potassium as a magic energy mineral, nutritionists note that potassium is one of many minerals and nutrients that contribute to overall energy—and that, while a potassium-rich banana, potato, or glass of apricot nectar all make good healthful snacks for active women, they are not miracle energy foods. Other sources of potassium are citrus fruits, tomatoes, and whole grains.

Sodium aids in digestion and in maintaining the body's proper fluid balance. In our modern society of processed and salted foods, deficiencies of sodium are exceedingly rare;

in fact, many health experts feel that our overindulgence in this mineral plays a role in the alarming rate of high blood pressure among Americans. Today, it's difficult to eat any type of prepared—canned, frozen, marinated—foods or condiments without taking in adequate salt.

Sulfur helps to maintain shiny hair and smooth, toned skin. Most of us get adequate sulfur in our diets by eating basic foods—meat, fish, legumes, nuts, eggs, and cabbage.

SMART HABITS

Today, most women are interested not only in eating for health and weight maintenance but also in eating for energy, to give us the extra edge we need to keep up with the busy lives that most of us lead. Here are some key suggestions to help ensure that you get a balanced array of the nutrients you need for health and energy, and that can keep your mood and energy in high gear:

Start with breakfast. Nutritionists now believe that breakfast is the most important meal of the day, from an energy and nutrition point of view. It literally starts your day with an energy boost and gives you a head start in getting your daily nutrients. The smartest breakfast, say experts, does not consist of a sweet roll and caffeine-laden coffee, or the eggs and bacon, toast and butter that we grew up on. The wise choice now is whole-wheat toast or whole-grain cereal, fruit, skim milk or low-fat cheese, plus, if you want, a cup of coffee, preferably decaffeinated.

Substitute herbs and spices for salt. Your food will taste better and your health will benefit. You'll also be less likely to retain water, not only in your body but in vulnerable facial areas such as under eyes and around jowls, where water retention leads to a bloated look.

Don't overindulge in alcohol. Not only can it show up in your face in the form of broken blood vessels but it can cause bloodshot eyes and less than fresh-looking skin. It is also high in empty calories that put on weight quickly. Keep your drinking to a minimum.

Don't overeat. Overeating taxes the body to the point at which it rebels; learning to eat smaller amounts of food means you don't have to deprive yourself of any favorites but you'll get less stomach upset and fewer extra (usually unneeded) calories.

Beware that food cravings are often habits, not nutritional needs. When you feel as if you have to have a chocolate bar, try doing something else instead—exercising, or snacking on a handful of raisins and nuts. This will satisfy your sugar craving.

Make desserts special-occasion foods. While dermatologists no longer feel that chocolate or sugar are the cause of skin problems, the weight gain that results from regularly eating rich desserts is not flattering to anyone. And skin that is once stretched to accommodate excess weight can lose its firmness for good. Instead, substitute fruit, cheese, and crackers for rich or sugary desserts, eating cakes or cookies only on special occasions.

WATER
Skin and Health Source

Water is nature's original beauty treatment, keeping our skin supple, smooth, and soft and helping to maintain internal and external health. The simplest thing any woman can do to improve her overall health and well-being, as well as the texture and tone of her skin, is to start drinking more water *now*.

A good daily guide is to consume eight or nine 8-ounce glasses every day. Watch beverages with caffeine; although they do contain water, the caffeine acts as a diuretic, robbing the body of fluids rather than supplementing them.

How does water help to maintain health and skin tone? To begin with, every cell in our bodies requires water for its essential structure and function. Water is the body's digestive solvent, moving food through the digestive tract, carrying fuel to the cells, and carrying away wastes. In addition, water acts as a lubricant between cells, blood vessels, joints, and internal organs. Our body temperature is maintained at a constant level thanks to our internal fluid balance and the processes of breathing and perspiration.

The texture of a woman's skin is a good indication of water's restorative powers. The truth is that the skin receives its essential moisture from the inside out; there is really no way to bring water to the skin from the outside as effectively. What moisturizing creams and lotions do is help to hold the water in the cells of the skin by preventing evaporation on the skin's surface. Without sufficient moisture—and the help of a "barrier" lotion or cream—the skin becomes flat, dull, and dehydrated, emphasizing the obviousness of fine surface lines and creases. Water "pumped" from within and kept from evaporating plumps up cells and gives the illusion of filling in tiny, dry surface lines.

CRASH DIETS
An Enemy of Skin and Health

It is estimated that as many as 60 million Americans are overweight—and that women are much more likely than men to experience weight problems. Just about every woman has at one point or another promised to start a diet "tomorrow"—a day that seemingly never really arrives!

The first thing every woman who wants to shed excess pounds needs to know: Most diets that promise to work very fast end very fast too, with the unhappy result that you gain back as much as or more than you've lost. The only way to become a slimmer woman for life is to start living like one; studies show that women who manage to maintain a steady healthful body weight are more physically active and eat less than their heavy-set counterparts.

A wise dieter will look for a balanced eating plan that includes no fewer than 1,200 calories a day (unless you're being monitored closely by a physician, never go on a diet lower in calories than this, regardless of how safe the diet book or article claims the diet to be). Beware of diets that center on a single food or require elaborate changes from your usual way of eating; you'll be less likely to stick with it. A safe, realistic expectation for weight loss, say nutritionists, is no more than 2 to 3 pounds per week; any more than that and the diet is probably dangerous to your health. (*Never* start any low-calorie eating plan without your doctor's approval, especially if you have a history of medical problems or are over thirty-five, pregnant, or breast-feeding.)

Avoiding crash diets not only makes weight-loss much more likely, it can also help to maintain the youthful look of your skin. Along with putting excessive strain on the heart and overall metabolism, crash dieting—especially repeatedly—takes a toll on your skin's tone and appearance. Gaining and losing weight quickly can cause a loss of moisture in skin tissue, literally stretching the skin and making it sag, bag, and wrinkle, especially when skin is restretched repeatedly by lifelong "yo-yo" dieting. In an effort to promote quick weight lose many diet plans are low in fluid intake and fats, both crucial to maintaining a healthy-looking complexion.

The best dieting advice I can offer to any woman, from the standpoint of a healthy heart and lungs, good circulation, and youthful-looking skin: Choose a body "size" best suited to nature's design for you early in adulthood and make a worthwhile commitment to maintaining it. Keeping your weight in a steady, attractive, healthy range will benefit your overall appearance, your long-term health, and your complexion.

If you do need to lose weight, do so gradually. Your goals should be to change your eating habits for life—that's the only way you'll be able to maintain a new, lower weight. And the latest research shows it will be much better for your overall health in the long run.

161

13

The Great Shape-Up

Today, the phrase *active woman* describes just about all of us. Whether we pursue jogging, tennis, aerobic dance, skiing, or gymnastics, there's no doubt we're moving, working our bodies, and working up a sweat more than our mothers and grandmothers would have ever believed possible.

The benefits of physical activity can be seen in the shape of women's bodies today and—the "unseen" but definite advantage—in our health and general well-being. Research suggests that exercise does much more than build strong, lean bodies; it also helps to prevent heart disease; fight obesity, high blood pressure, and diabetes; and release built-up tension and anxiety. Exercise is the best preventive health step a woman can take—and it is something that a woman can begin at just about any age.

EXERCISE
Skin Energizer?

Some of the other positive side effects of living an active life are increased blood flow and improved circulation—benefits that some experts theorize make an important difference in the look of an exerciser's skin. Some doctors suggest that the increased metabolism that comes from exercise, and that makes it possible to burn off extra fat and calories, may also speed up nourishment of skin cells, helping the skin to renew itself faster and to keep itself looking younger. These experts feel that the same "stimulation" of the body's energy and self-fueling processes is evident in exercises' impact on the skin.

Until all the research studies are completed, it's impossible to guarantee that working out for four hours this week will make your skin look "X years younger" next summer. But one thing is certain: Many women who take up the exercise habit notice a change in their attitude, in their thinking about their appearance that translates into feeling better about themselves. And feeling good about yourself, having confidence in your abilities, and taking pleasure in your life is the best "antiaging" formula your complexion can have. What's more, taking up a new exercise program, feeling more vibrant, and being more active is also likely to add a wonderful "glow" to your complexion—which may be the most visible exercise benefit of all.

WORKING UP A SWEAT— AND TAKING IT OFF

The saying used to be, "men sweat, women glow." In past years, no woman would admit to, let alone aim for, working up a sweat. Today, we know that sweating is healthy—that it indicates our exercise routines are working, that we are burning off fat and building up muscle.

But sweat, if not removed from the skin's surface, can wreak havoc on a woman's complexion. Perspiration is a mixture of water, body salts, and acidic waste products—materials that can clog pores, irritate sensitive skin, and lead to unattractive breakouts if skin is not cleansed regularly, *before* and *after* a workout. Also a must for an active woman: keeping everything that comes into contact with your skin during exercise—your clothes, your hair, your sweatband—as clean and bacteria-free as possible.

Although just about any soap will cleanse sweat off your body and underarm areas without causing much of a problem, the skin of your face is far more delicate than other body areas and requires more gentle cleansing. Never use a deodorant soap on your face—it strips away much-needed skin oils and will lead to dryness and irritation. Instead, use a gentle cleansing cream to remove all makeup *before* exercising and to cleanse away perspiration afterward.

Working out while wearing full face makeup is, undoubtedly, the *worst* thing you can do for your complexion. Perspiration is the natural cooling process for your body; blocking the evaporation of sweat by sealing the skin with makeup interferes with this process. And, even worse, when perspiration mixes with makeup, it increases the chance of an adverse skin reaction to your makeup. So, regardless of whom you expect to meet at the gym or health club, limit your makeup to lip gloss and, if you insist, waterproof mascara.

SKIN FITNESS
Cleansing Plus Protection

Here is a basic skin-fitness routine for every exerciser, plus specific advice for the most common sports.

Before Exercising. Cleanse your face and neck, where skin is most sensitive, with a gentle cleansing lotion plus water (if you're wearing makeup, use a creamy cleanser to remove it first). Rinse well with splashes of warm-to-cool (not hot) water. If you have long hair or bangs, tie your hair back or use a headband to keep hair off your face. Sweat "trapped" against skin by hair is a common cause of postexercise skin breakouts, so always keep rubber bands and barrettes on hand.

Don't use a harsh astringent before exercising. Your natural skin oils can actually act as a buffer between the acid content of perspiration and sensitive skin layers. So save the astringent or toner for postworkout cleansing.

Exercising Outdoors. Always apply a moisturizing sunscreen—whether your skin is oily or dry. The sun is the most dangerous element we encounter, so always take time to protect your skin before heading outdoors. If you'll be exercising in cold or windy conditions, let the moisturizing sunscreen "set" for five minutes, then reapply another skin-protecting layer. In summer, always use the highest sun protection factor you can find—which means at least SPF 15 (today, you can find lotions as protective as SPF 23 to 30+, some formulated especially for the face).

Exercising Indoors. Gyms usually have a high humidity factor. Even though this may feel a bit uncomfortable at first, be thankful, for the humidity will "hold" moisture in your skin and lessen the irritating and drying effects of perspiration (if you have a history of breathing problems or allergies, however, check with your doctor before working out in a hot, humid gym). Unless the air inside the room you'll be working out in is very dry, start your workout with freshly cleansed skin and apply no moisturizing oils or creams. If you work out in a very dry, overheated city apartment, consider installing a humidifier, or apply a lightweight moisturizer before exercising.

During Exercise. If you perspire heavily, keep a towel handy to pat—not rub—some of the sweat away. If

165

your skin is very oily and prone to breakouts of any kind, arm yourself with several cotton balls dipped in cleansing lotion to wipe the perspiration off your face. If it's a hot day, also keep a tube of sunscreen handy and reapply it every fifteen minutes or so; the second that it takes will not interrupt the pace of your exercise session and will be of real benefit to the long-term health and youthful appearance of your skin.

Postworkout. Finish every exercise session with a cool-down, doing several minutes of stretching and gentle flexibility-boosting moves to calm pumped-up muscles and give your body a chance to rid your muscles of excess fluids and wastes. (Contrary to what most of us were led to believe, the biggest boost to flexibility is achieved by doing your stretching *after* aerobics, when your muscles are truly warmed up.) After your cooldown, head for the shower and turn up the warm (not too hot or cold) water. Don't overlook all-important cleansing spots such as shoulders and back, where sweat can pool under clothing and cause breakouts later on. If you like the tingly clean feel of a cleansing sponge, body brush, or loofah, now is the time to use one—but never on blemished or irritated skin areas, and never in a harsh rubbing motion. Never use a loofah or deodorant soap on your face; instead, use a cleansing lotion formulated for your skin type, or if your skin can tolerate it, a grainy cleanser.

Shampoo your hair after *every* exercise session; this is the time when it's a special pleasure to use a scented shampoo. For last-minute invigoration, try a cool head-to-toe rinse-off, then wrap your body in a big, fluffy towel and pat—don't rub—skin dry,

dusting your skin with a fragrant talc afterward. As the final step, lavish a rich, creamy moisturizer (perhaps a body cream in your favorite fragrance) on legs, arms, shoulders, and elbows, plus a lighter moisturizer on face and neck. Then it's time to reach for a tall, cool glass of water or fruit juice (or a mineral water and lime juice "cocktail" spiced with a sprig of fresh mint) to replenish needed body fluids. And take a few minutes to put your feet up and congratulate yourself for an effort well spent.

Remember that where there's perspiration, there's evaporation—and loss of vital body fluids. Since more than 50 percent of our bodies is made up of water, the water you lose during exercise needs to be replenished. Give your body a head start by drinking one or two glasses of water, fruit juice, or unsweetened vegetable juice before exercise, and take a water or juice break (try fruit juice diluted with an equal part of water) midway through your workout, more often if it's a particularly hot day. Even the most highly trained marathon runners stop for liquid refreshment at water stations placed throughout the course. Follow their example and don't wait until you feel thirsty to replenish fluids; our bodies' thirst mechanisms actually lag behind our need for fluids and don't kick in until we're getting dangerously low. Drink *before* you become thirsty and you'll have more endurance and a safe, more pleasant workout.

WHAT TO WEAR

Today, workout clothes are being worn not only to the gym but to give a woman an active image while shopping, heading for a casual date, or even simply walking the dog. Yet when it comes to maintaining skin health, the clothes you wear for exercise must fit their function as well as they fit your body shape. Here are some points to remember when choosing workout gear, whatever activity you choose:

Wear loose-fitting, natural-fiber clothing whenever possible. Although you may want to show off your shape while you're working out, don't wear clothing that constricts movement or that is made of fibers that don't breathe. All-nylon leotards, for example, can keep perspiration from evaporating and cause acne-type breakouts or rashes; the best leotards to wear are made from all-cotton fabrics or mostly cotton blends or from high-tech fibers, such as polypropylene, that allow sweat to evaporate.

Keep your sweat clothes sweat-free. Launder your workout gear after each wearing, not only to feel fresher but to keep bacteria away from skin's surface. Don't forget headbands, wristbands, and cover-ups as well as leotards, shorts, T-shirts, and jogging suits. If you're hiking or camping, watch for skin inflammation caused by an ill-adjusted backpack or straps rubbing against sweat-moist skin.

Watch for chafe points. Don't buy activewear that is too tight or, conversely, that has too much excess fabric at the skin's vulnerable points of contact—under arms, between legs, at the waistband. Most exercise experts recommend that a woman wear a bra while doing any type of exercise that involves up-and-down or jarring movement, such as aerobic dance, jogging, or jumping rope. However, choose a bra that not only fits well but doesn't contain any metal or heavy plastic hooks or closures, as sweat can pool under these areas and cause skin irritation. Likewise, always wear all-cotton underwear while exercising. If skin irritation or chafing does occur, relieve the itchiness with cornstarch-and-water compresses (mix ½ cup cornstarch with 1 pint cool-to-lukewarm water). Any irritation or rash that does not disappear within a few days, or that grows worse the second day rather than better, should be checked by a dermatologist rather than self-treated.

SPORT SPECIFICS

The general skin care and equipment advice outlined above applies to every woman and every type of physical activity. Here are some more considerations to take into account for specific types of exercises:

Aerobic Dance. Aerobic dance has become increasingly popular because it is a way to make exercise fun. Some skin protective advice:

• Never wear makeup to class. Perspiration and makeup combine to produce skin irritation, rashes, and acne breakouts—so do your skin a favor. While some women think that just wearing eye makeup is a good compromise, be aware that eye makeup can run with heavy perspiration (and this goes even for the supposedly waterproof kind), which not only looks unattractive but, if makeup gets into your eyes, can be irritating.

• Try to leave a window slightly ajar when exercising. Ventilation will help sweat to evaporate off skin's surface, and decrease the chances of exercisers becoming overheated.

• Always keep your hair off of your face during aerobics class. Even if your hair is cut short, use a headband to keep stray pieces off your forehead and cheeks.

• If your exercise routine includes a good deal of jumping up and down, pay special attention to your feet after class. After showering, apply talcum powder between toes and add extra moisturizing cream to feet (soles as well as tops) to smooth rough skin.

• Never skip your postworkout shower. You'll want to remove perspiration from skin's surface right away to prevent its irritating effects—and to cleanse sweat off your scalp and hair, as well. To give your skin a postworkout treat, keep a fragranced moisturizer or talc in your locker to apply after showering, and lavish moisturizer on rough spots—feet, knees, elbows.

Tennis, Squash, and Racquetball. Before and after every game:

• Cleanse your face thoroughly before a game, following up with a moisturizer.

• If you're playing outdoors, wear a sunscreen, even on a cloudy day. And apply an eye cream and lip "screen" to provide moisture and protection for these delicate skin areas. Wear a sun visor and sunglasses so you don't squint—an often unacknowledged cause of later wrinkles.

• If you wear sweatbands or wristbands, launder them in a gentle detergent after every game.

• Take a break between sets to cleanse your face (carry cotton balls moistened with water-souble cleanser or an astringent) and to drink a tall glass of water. If you're outdoors, use this time, too, to reapply sunblock.

• Follow every game with a cool-

down and a shower, applying moisturizer to body and face afterward (don't forget rough spots like hands and soles).

Swimming. This is one of the best all-around exercises, but it can also be rough on the complexion, so certain skin-care tips are key . . .

• If you swim outdoors, always apply a waterproof sunscreen SPF 15 before you step outdoors. Sunlight not only penetrates water, but can be reflected off the water's surface and onto your skin for a double whammy effect. Reapply waterproof sunscreen every twenty minutes or so for continued protection—and try to get out of the sun and under an umbrella or other shady area when you come out of the water.

• Be aware that chlorine and salt water can both have a drying effect on skin (and that the chlorine level in many indoor pools is much higher than in outdoor swimming pools). Before you take the plunge, cover your skin with a protective moisturizer if you'll be indoors, a moisturizing sunscreen formula if you're headed outside.

• Remember that your hair is also vulnerable to chlorine damage. Ideally, you should wear a bathing cap. The second best move is applying a conditioning lotion to wet hair before swimming and rinsing hair well with clear water as soon as you get out of the pool.

• Shower immediately after swiming, even if it's just a clear water total-body rinse-off. Take advantage of the outdoor showers found at many pools and beaches—but don't overlook the need to rinse your face and hair as well as your body and to reapply sunscreen from head to foot.

• When you get finished with your swimming for the day, take a shower and use a gentle, creamy body cleanser to remove all traces of chlorine or salt from skin, and a moisturizing shampoo to rinse away chlorine or salt from hair and scalp. Finish up with a gentle hair conditoner; postshower, apply a scented body cream and talcum powder.

Skiing. This is the perfect winter sport—but following certain guidelines is essential:

• Always be sure that your skin is thoroughly dry before you head outdoors. Damp skin is especially vulnerable to the hazards of cold, wind, and sun and is prone to chapping and cracking.
• Use an SPF 15 sunscreen or opaque (zinc oxide) sunblock whatever the weather. Clouds may block some of the sun's rays, but they do allow others to get through—and skiing's high-altitude location means that the potential for sun damage is multiplied.
• Wear ski goggles with dark lenses that block ultraviolet rays to protect your eyes and the delicate skin surrounding them. Preventing the need to squint will not only make skiing more comfortable but will help to prevent the tell-tale lines around the eyes and on the forehead that characterize skiers' sun damage.
• Wear a lip balm that is formulated with emollients and suncreen.
• If your hands tend to become chapped and dry in cold weather, apply an emollient hand cream, allowing it to absorb into skin a few minutes before putting on your gloves.
• When you come indoors, avoid the skin "shock" of immediately sitting in front of a red-hot fireplace (in fact, recent skin research indicates direct heat may intensify the wrinkling aftereffects of sun exposure). Instead, take a few minutes to cleanse your skin gently with a mild cleansing lotion and lukewarm water. If you take a shower, apply a rich moisturizing lotion to face and body. Once your skin is thoroughly lubricated and acclimatized to the warm indoor temperatures, then you can go sit by the fire.

Water-Skiing and Boating. These are favorite summer pastimes. Cool sea breezes can be deceptive, however, making us forget that our skin is getting a great deal of exposure to the sun. What to do:

• Be aware that salt spray, plus sun reflection off of the water and sand, can intensify the drying and long-term damaging effects of the sun. "Arm" your skin with the defenses of an SPF 15 waterproof sunscreen that contains rich moisturizing ingredients, and reapply every hour if you're spending a good deal of the time in the water.
• Pack a bag containing sun block, moisturizer, lip balm, eye cream, and—for refreshment—a spritzer of cool mineral water to spray on skin if you get too hot.
• For extra protection, wear sunglasses and a hat while on the boat; always reapply sunscreen as soon as you get out of the water.
• When you head for a postboating shower, apply a heavy moisturizer *beforehand*, then reapply afterward. Pay special attention to sun-tinged spots—nose, cheeks, tops of shoulders, elbows.

TAKING THE HEAT
Sauna and Steam Room Smarts

For many women, a postexercise session in the sauna or steam room is wonderfully relaxing, a perfect way to wind down after a strenuous workout or game of tennis or golf. While saunas and steam rooms may feel relaxing, however, they need to be approached cautiously, not only from the point of view of protecting your skin but, more important, of safeguarding your health. Anyone who has any sort of medical problem—a heart or circulatory condition or any condition requiring medication—or anyone who is pregnant should never go into a sauna or steam room without checking with a physician first. If you have highly sensitive skin—are pale-complexioned, blond, tend to develop broken capillaries or eczema, or sunburn very easily—you should also skip any treatment involving a great deal of heat on your skin.

Remove all of your makeup before going into a sauna or steam room. It is also a good idea to apply a creamy conditioner to your hair to help prevent it from becoming too dry. To prevent heat-induced dehydration, keep your steam or sauna sessions short—say, no more than five minutes. Drink a glass of water before going in for a sauna or steam, and another glass afterward. If your skin is dry, wash your face after exercising and apply a rich lubricant to face and neck, blotting off the excess and leaving a thin film of moisturizer to provide skin protection. When you come out of the steam room or sauna, use cool-water splashes plus a very gentle cleanser to clean your skin, and follow up with a rich application of a moisturizer appropriate to your skin type.

THE BOTTOM LINE
Don't Overdo It

The most important thing to remember about any exercise routine is the importance of moderation; any excessive muscle soreness or joint pain should be a signal to stop exercising, take a few days off, and let your body recover. At every exercise level—professional as well as beginning—injury can be caused by carelessness or overdoing it. Professional athletes, of course, often have the luxury of a masseuse or physical therapist waiting in the locker room after each game, but every exerciser can create her own postworkout relaxation with a little bit of effort ahead of time. Here are my recipes for after-exercise self-recovery:

Blister Balm

To smooth feet before or after sports, mash 2 figs in a small ceramic bowl; blend in 1 tablespoon honey. Apply to sore spots on feet; leave on 20 minutes. Rinse off with lukewarm water; follow with a rich moisturizing cream (to avoid skin sensitivity, chose a fragrance-free moisturizer).

Postplay Foot Soak

Fill a plastic tub with warm water plus 1 cup Epsom salts. Soak feet for 15 minutes; pat dry with a clean, fluffy towel. Holding your toes, bend and rotate your ankle inward and outward several times; repeat with the other foot. Make a fist and, using a gentle circular motion, massage the sole of your foot; repeat with other foot. Starting at the toes, use both hands to massage the entire foot slowly, working back to the heel and up to the ankle; repeat, then do twice on other foot. Take each toe and gently pull upward and twist around gently. *Apply a rich moisturizer, massaging it into the skin from ankles to toes.*

Hair Toner

To use as a final hair and scalp rinse after shampooing: Combine ½ cup white wine vinegar, ½ cup distilled water, and 2 tablespoons chamomile flowers (or loose chamomile tea). Boil for 15 minutes, then strain. Allow to cool; use as an after-shampoo refresher. (Can be prepared ahead of time and kept in the refrigerator.)

Skin Primer

The perfect postexercise skin refresher to have on hand in the refrigerator: Combine 1 tablespoon rosemary, 3 tablespoons chamomile flowers (or loose chamomile tea), and 3 cups distilled water. Boil for 15 minutes. Strain; refrigerate. Use a cotton ball to pat onto skin after perspiring. (Can be put in a small plastic bottle and toted along to the tennis court or exercise class.)

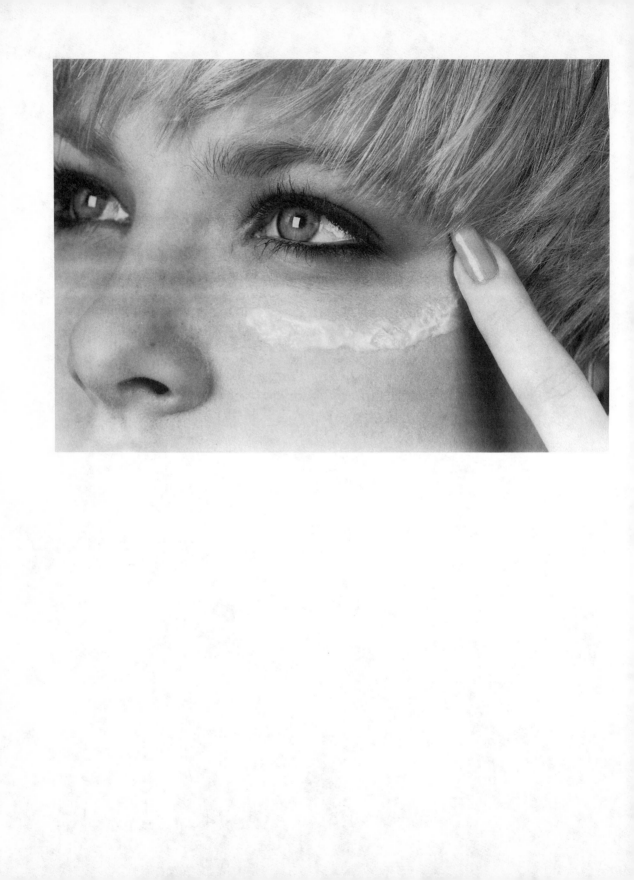

14

The Eyes Have It

Our eyes are our most expressive features—the "mirrors of the soul," as they've been called. Since Cleopatra's time, women have used makeup to accent the shape and size of their eyes; in more modern times, we've come to know that the skin around the eyes is the most delicate skin of our bodies. We've also learned that taking care to protect the eye area from sun, wind, and irritating cosmetics can help to keep the skin of this area looking smooth and young.

THE EYES DESERVE IT
Protection

It's important to realize that the skin around your eyes can react to wind, sun exposure, too much heat, and the dryness of air conditioning, as well as the irritation caused by perfumed cosmetics or the effort to rub away eye makeup. Because this skin contains few oil glands, the subtle signs of aging often show up first in fine lines and wrinkles around the eyes.

The first step is to protect your eyes from sun exposure by wearing sunglasses that shield against ultraviolet light (these glasses can also protect the eyes themselves against damage caused by sunlight—the impact of which many experts believe contributes to cataracts). By blocking out the sun's glare, you'll prevent squinting—the prime cause of the formation of lines and wrinkles around the eyes. Ask an optometrist to recommend a pair of sunglasses that block both UVA and UVB radiation. Remember to wear sunglasses in the winter, too—sunlight reflected off of the snow can cause a condition known as "snow blindness," in which eyes become painfully red and irritated and you have difficulty seeing clearly when you return indoors.

For additional year-round protection, I also recommend applying a sunscreen around the eyes—but you must be especially careful to choose a product that is formulated not to "creep" into the eyes themselves. (Be particularly careful not to get sunscreen products into your eyes, as the ingredients in these products can sting terribly. If this should happen, rinse your eyes repeatedly with cool water, then lie down with your eyes closed for several minutes before going outdoors.)

The second, equally important, line of defense against wrinkles around your eyes is to start wearing an eye cream no later than age twenty-five. Again, choose one that will moisturize and lubricate, but will not "creep" into the eyes.

Eye-area moisturizers are commonly found in three forms: cream, gel, and oil. I believe that the cream formula is the best—it slowly penetrates into the skin, is nongreasy, and stays where it is applied (which means it won't seep into and irritate eyes as the day goes on). Oils are far greasier, as their name implies, and tend to sit on the surface of the skin rather than being absorbed into the skin; and gels can feel a little "tight" and irritating on this most delicate skin area. *Never* use a moisturizer that is not specifically labeled as safe for use around the eyes, or one that contains perfume; even the slightest hint of perfume in a formula can cause puffiness and irritation. Any eye cream should be applied with care—patted, not rubbed, into the skin area just below the lashes. If you're applying eye cream under your makeup, always apply it a few minutes ahead of time, to allow the cream to be absorbed by the skin before you start applying concealer or foundation.

For additional skin smoothing, a facialist may apply a gentle creamy mask to the skin around, but not quite next to, the eyes—a warm paraffin mask, for example. This can help to "plump up" fine lines and give the skin a fresher, younger appearance.

If you apply a facial mask at home, be especially careful to leave a "ring" of bare skin around the eyes; you don't want any cream or mask to seep into the eyes, as this can cause irritation.

GENTLE CARING
Wrinkle Protection

In addition to choosing the proper protection for the delicate eye area, you must be especially careful in applying or removing cosmetics in the eye area.

Makeup Application. I always recommend using soft, sponge-tipped applicators to apply eye shadows, and choosing only soft, easily smudgeable eye pencils and crayons. Never pull or tug at the skin around the eyes as you apply makeup; this increases the chances of the skin in this area "stretching" and wrinkling.

When applying mascara, always be careful to avoid getting it in the eyes; the color pigments in mascara can build up in the inner tissue of the eyelids and cause infection or allergy over time. I recommend avoiding waterproof mascara formulas, as these contain ingredients that are chemically similar to glue, which means they take a great deal of rubbing to remove thoroughly. If you wear contact lenses, never use a mascara that claims to lengthen or thicken lashes:

The fibrous material in these mascaras can come off the lashes and cause irritation and, in some cases, fuse with soft lenses, making them unwearable. (Apply makeup after putting in lenses.)

Eye Makeup Removal. Always use a compressed cotton pad and a liquid eye makeup remover to rinse away eye makeup gently; never use an ordinary cotton ball (the fuzz can get into eyes) or a tissue (which can be too harsh on delicate eye-area skin). You will need to use several cotton pads to remove makeup thoroughly—this is perfectly fine, so long as you are gentle each time in simply patting the remover onto the skin around your eyes. What is essential is that you always remove all eye makeup before going to sleep to prevent color pigments from "creeping" into the eye area and building up under the skin of the lids. In addition, mascara left on lashes is a prime cause of lash breakage, a problem that I see very often in young women in my salon. It's wiser to take a few extra minutes before you go to sleep at night to remove all of your makeup, regardless of how tired you are, if you want to protect the look of your skin later on. If you wear contact lenses, of course, always be sure to remove your lenses *before* taking off your eye makeup.

EYEBROWS
Perfect Proportion

It is a lucky few women—Brooke Shields among them—who seem to have been born with perfectly shaped, perfectly proportioned eyebrows. For the rest of us, a *little* targeted plucking can help to produce neater, but still natural-looking brows.

The problem: Too many women get carried away with a tweezer, producing too-thin, unnatural-looking eyebrows.

To outline the proper proportion of your brows, rest an orange stick against the outside of your nose on the left side and hold it in a perfectly straight vertical line. Where the stick intersects the browline is where your brow should start. Keeping the lower end of the orange stick against your left nostril, slant the stick until it crosses the outer corner of your left eye. That is a natural-looking endpoint for your brow. To size up your right eyebrow, repeat these same steps on the other eye.

To tweeze your eyebrows like a professional means to remove very few hairs, just enough to shape the brows and leave them looking natural. I prefer a pointed-tip tweezer, because it provides me with the most precision, but some of you may find angled-tip tweezers easier to use (don't use blunt-tip tweezers, they remove too many hairs at once). Always sterilize the tweezers by wiping them with alcohol before each use to prevent skin irritation or infection, and gently stretch the skin of the brows to minimize discomfort. Pluck one hair at a time from underneath the brow line, gently pulling the hair in the direction of growth. If in doubt, undertweeze; better to have to touch up your brows the next day than to suffer with overly tweezed brows for weeks. If you want to emphasize your brows before going out at night, dot a soft brown pencil onto skin, then smudge and blend for a natural-looking result.

If, like many women, you find it difficult—or painful—to tweeze your own eyebrows, you might consider having it done professionally while you have a facial or other treatment at a beauty salon. In many cases, estheticians use wax to remove hairs between the brows, or to neaten the line above or below the brows. Care should be taken to avoid the spreading or dripping of wax anywhere near the eyes themselves, of course, and waxing of the brows should be done only by a professional, *never* at home. To soothe the skin afterward, a chamomile or buttermilk mask may be applied. The skin may look slightly pink afterward for anywhere from a half- to three hours, but if irritation persists you should not have waxing done again, as your skin is too sensitive. (For more information on grooming your brows see chapter 8.)

GETTING THE RED OUT
Coping with Irritated Eyes

Nothing is more disconcerting than looking in the mirror in the morning and seeing puffy, bloodshot eyes—or feeling as if your eyes are so itchy or grainy that you can't stop rubbing them. If this happens, the only solution is to close your eyes and let their natural self-cleaning mechanism—tears—go to work, or to help the process along by using a tear substitute solution available without prescription in pharmacies (examples of this type of artificial-tear solution are Tears Plus or Tears Naturale). Try to avoid the use of commercial eye-whitening drops; these are actually vasoconstrictors, which work by constricting the blood vessels within the eyes. Over time, according to ophthalmologists, your eyes can become dependent on such drops, with the result being *more* redness and *more* eye irritation unless you continue to use the drops, thus creating a vicious cycle.

Here are some common causes—and solutions—for irritated eyes, with advice from leading ophthalmologists:

Summer eyes. In the summer, the glare of the sun, plus exposure to chlorine and salt water, often produces eye redness and irritation. The best protection is wearing ultraviolet-screening sunglasses whenever you're outdoors and never looking directly into the sun. When swimming, it's a good idea always to wear goggles to keep chlorine or salt from coming into contact with the delicate corneal tissue of the eyes. Another preventive step: Never wear eye makeup when you're swimming or exercising outdoors; water and perspiration can "wash" the makeup into eyes, resulting in irritation.

Winter eyes. As I mentioned earlier, it's especially important to wear ultraviolet-screening sunglasses in winter, when the bright reflection of sunlight off of snow can create a painful condition called "snow blindness." Other dangers posed by cold, windy outdoor environments include dryness of the cornea surface, a condition that can be prevented by applying a few drops of artificial-tear solution into eyes before or after spending a great deal of time outdoors. If you can't avoid spending time in a dry, heated room, use a humidifier whenever possible.

Airplane eyes. The dry conditions inside an airplane cabin can exacerbate "dry eye syndrome," in which tears evaporate from the eye surface and redness and irritation develops. Here again, the best protection is to use an artificial-tear solution, apply-ing one or two drops before you board the plane, then every hour or so—or more often, if eyes feel itchy and irritated—after take-off. If you can manage to remove eye makeup, especially mascara, before you use the tear solution, all the better.

"Smoke gets in your eyes." This is more than the title of an old song—it's often the reality in a crowded restaurant, office, or party. If you're going to be in an environment that you know will be very smoky—and you are prone to irritation—try to plan on taking several breaks away from the smoky environment. Bring along an artificial-tear solution and apply a drop or two to each eye during this break. When you get home, try to take a few minutes to lie down and close your eyes to allow some of the irritation to dissipate.

TV eyes. Watching television in a dark room—or spending hours staring at a computer monitor—can cause eyestrain or irritation. The solution, say experts, is to be sure that any time you are looking at a video-type screen, the lighting in the room is planned to reduce glare and be "kind" to your eyesight. If you find yourself squinting at the screen, that's a sure sign that you need to adjust the intensity or placement of lighting. More and more computers are now made with nonglare screens; if your employer hasn't bought one of them, you can obtain a similar "eye-kind" image by purchasing a see-through plastic glare protector that fits right over the computer screen. Whatever type of monitor you use, adjust the contrast carefully to reduce glare, and take frequent breaks to minimize discomfort not only for eyes but for your arms, shoulders, and neck muscles as well.

GLASSES
Form Plus Function

Choosing the right glasses begins, of course, with a conversation with an ophthalmologist or optometrist, who, along with providing you with the proper eyeglass prescription, can let you know whether there is a particular type of eyeglass frame that makes the most sense for your needs. After that, care should be taken to choose glasses that are flattering to your face shape, hair color, skin tone, and the type of image you want to project—classic, sophisticated, or trendy.

Glasses and Makeup. This combination has always been tricky. After all, glasses function as a form of eye "makeup" on their own—but today, the guidelines are less a matter of how much eye makeup you wear than how it's applied. After all, eye makeup in general is more subtle now than ever. A woman who wears glasses should be aware of the fact that, regardless of her prescription, glasses will usually exaggerate the impact of any eye makeup you apply—so apply colors with the lightest of hands and spend time blending the makeup carefully. In general, what you want from eye makeup today is emphasis on eye shape and size—not an artificial-looking recoloring of the skin around your eyes.

Where you need to be especially careful is in the application of mascara. Nothing is less attractive than the look of clumped-up, overmascara-ed lashes seen through the lenses of prescription glasses, or the look of lashes that brush up against the lenses themselves. A general guideline: Apply a single coat of mascara, let it dry, then if you feel you need more, apply a *touch* of mascara only to lash ends. Wait a minute; then use a small lash brush to remove all excess mascara.

If you wear tinted lenses, go especially light on eye makeup; choose neutral shades, or it will look as if you're wearing color on top of color. If you wear bifocals or very thick lenses, again, minimalism should be the rule—no eye liner, no harsh colored shadows. Instead, choose a simple neutral color (soft brown, brown-black, midnight gray or blue) and rim your eyes with a smudged soft line. Never extend the color beyond the frames of your lenses, and never apply an opaque line—you'll want to be able to see the tone of your skin through a soft smudge of color. For farsighted women, the biggest concern is that the lenses will exaggerrate the size of your eyes. Makeup should be soft, minimal, with attention to subtle coverage of undereye circles.

Glasses and Eyebrows. The question of whether eyebrows and glasses should line up or cover each other has been debated among makeup experts for years. The current thought is that, rather than trying to line your glasses up precisely on top of your brows, it makes more sense to have the line of your glasses either above or below your brow line, since the effort to align the two precisely usually ends up with snatches of brow seen through the lens.

EYE Q'S
Questions and Answers

Here are some questions that I am often asked by clients in my salon:

Q: I often wake up with puffy eyes in the morning. What causes this? What should I do?

A: Eye puffiness is often caused by fluid retention that occurs while we sleep, and often "cures" itself as a result of gravity after we are up and about for a few hours. One wise preventive step is to eat a diet that is low in salt (or sodium) to minimize the chances of fluid retention. Another good idea is to sleep with your head elevated about 8 inches or so—roughly the thickness of two pillows. To speed up the disappearance of puffiness, try cool compresses of a mixture of milk and water, or cool chamomile tea. Lie down, apply the compresses to closed eyes, and relax for a few minutes. If you must leave the house before you can use compresses, apply undereye concealer in a shade one tone lighter than your skin color (don't overdo the concealer; you'll just get an unnatural-looking result).

Proof that this advice works: A stunning young actress who is a client of mine complained to me about puffiness under her eyes and said she was considering plastic surgery. I suggested she try using cool chamomile tea compresses for a few days first. She came back to my salon a few days later with a big smile on her face. "You've saved me thousands of dollars and weeks of recovery time," she said. "I tried the compresses and they worked wonders."

In some cases, of course, puffiness of the skin around the eyes is caused by allergies such as hay fever; recurrent eye puffiness that doesn't disappear over the course of the day should be brought to a doctor's attention. Puffy bags *under* the eyes may also actually be the result of an inherited accumulation of excess fatty tissue; in such cases, the problem can be cured only by plastic surgery.

Q: Can I sleep away dark circles under my eyes?

A: Dark circles under the eyes are actually caused by blood vessels lying close to the surface of the skin, which is an inherited problem. They can also be the result of shadows cast by "bags" of excess fat under the eyes (also an inherited problem). Dark circles can be made more obvious by lack of sleep, so getting an extra hour or so of sleep can help to minimize them, although sleep is not a cure.

Good makeup can help greatly to minimize dark undereye circles. Choose a concealer one tone *lighter* than your skin tone and apply it under your foundation. Another option that looks very natural on pale-toned complexions is to use a pinky-taupe-colored foundation and simply dot a little bit of the foundation on the undereye area, then apply your usual foundation and blend with your pinky or middle finger (always be especially gentle in applying and blending makeup around your eyes). *Don't* use white concealer under any circumstances; it looks very unnatural.

Overconsumption of alcoholic beverages can exacerbate undereye circles by causing the blood vessels to dilate. During your menstrual period, you may also notice that blood vessels on the face become more noticeable, so a bit of extra care in applying your makeup may be wise.

Q: By the end of the day, my eyes feel dry and itchy—and the skin around them becomes puffy and blotchy. Any advice?

A: Overexposure to sun, wind, or the dry air found in many homes and offices can cause eyes to become dry and irritated. Concentration on your work can also contribute to the problem: When we stare intently at a piece of paper or computer screen, we often neglect to blink, which means we don't stimulate the eyes' natural release of soothing tears often enough.

Blinking your eyes regularly can help, as can literally closing your eyes once an hour for a few minutes (I often do this while I'm talking on the phone). If you work in an office with very dry air, consider asking for a humidifier—or invest in one yourself. If eyes become dry and irritated, a quick fix is to use a lubricating tears solution—*not*, though, the type of drops that claim to remove redness, as these contain harmful vasoconstrictors that can cause your eyes to have a "rebound" reaction and become more red and irritated over time.

If irritated eyes become a regular problem, consult an ophthalmologist, as this may be the symptom of a need for eyeglasses or another vision problem.

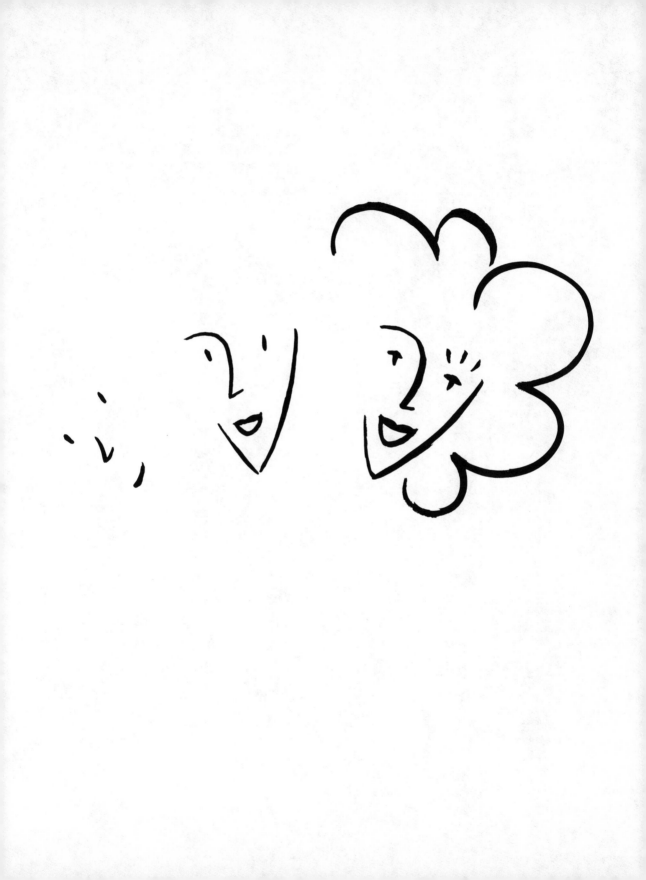

15

Modern Make-Up

American women have long had a love affair with makeup—and with good reason. Artfully applied, makeup can help to accent one's best features and flatter skin tone and hair color. What is also true, however, is that, like all good things, too much makeup looks unattractive, artificial, and out of fashion. Another consideration is choosing makeup in flattering colors and with a formula appropriate to your skin type to avoid the myriad skin problems that can result from simply using the wrong formulation.

In this chapter, I will give you guidelines for choosing, using, and evaluating cosmetics in a way that will help you to maintain healthy- and attractive-looking skin. This advice is based not only on my own years of experience but on conversations with expert makeup artists whose work has appeared in the pages of many national magazines. Remember that this advice is meant as a general introduction to the use of cosmetics; your personal taste, as well as your skill in applying makeup, will influence your choice of makeup as well.

FIRST CHOICE
The Skin-Makeup Match

The first topic in any discussion of makeup, for me, is the subject of skin type. Broadly speaking, as I've outlined in chapter 6, skin falls into three general categories: dry, oily, and combination (what is usually termed *normal* skin). Many makeup products such as foundations are available in these categories—but the specificity of these formulas varies greatly from one manufacturer to another. What is sold for "normal-to-oily" skin by company X may be twice as creamy

as the same type of formula from company Y. Which brings me to an important point: The best makeup choices are, unfortunately, often a matter of trial and error, of trying different products and then deciding which ones work best for you. There are, however, several points to be understood in shopping for and using any type of cosmetics:

Sample products before you buy them. The best way to test a cosmetic's compatibility with your skin is to wear it for a while. Only then can you tell whether your skin will feel irritated, or greasy, or "trapped" under a heavy mask as a result of wearing a particular foundation—or whether your eyes will feel puffy or watery when wearing a particular mascara. The best way to sample products is not by using the makeup testers found on department store counters; these open-to-the-air sample trays may be contaminated by other customers' fingers, by perfume sprayed into the air around them, or simply by dust settling into an open container. Also, your skin is usually not especially clean when you walk into a store in midafternoon, after walking around the city or being at your job for several hours. A far better way to sample products is by having a makeup application done first, by a professional makeup artist, whom you can make an appointment to see in a salon or department store or at some cosmetics counters. She or he will cleanse your skin and also cleanse any tools or products to be used in applying cosmetics to your face, and can offer you helpful advice in using makeup as well. Very often, the cost of these professional makeup applications will be redeemable, at least in part, in makeup products, so you will be getting what amounts to free advice and a free "trial" period of a day wearing the cosmetics.

Don't try too many new products all at once. Any woman who has suffered rashes or other skin problems in response to cosmetics in the past should be very careful in trying new products in the future. By limiting yourself to wearing one new product in any given week, you'll both protect yourself from the possibility of an intense reaction to a new product line and be able to isolate the cause of any skin response that occurs.

Consider wearing makeup and skin care products available from the same salon or company. Not only are these products formulated in a compatible manner—in other words, the foundation is made to slide on smoothly over the moisturizer, the powder doesn't cake up on top of the foundation—but you will have already had a "trial run" with many of the ingredients used in the cosmetics by wearing the skin lotions and using the cleansers. It's no secret that most companies use a basic group of ingredients that are found in their individual cosmetics as well as skin care products, so you'll be less likely to have a skin reaction to other makeup products made by that same company.

Check packages carefully before purchasing a cosmetic. I am not trying to be an alarmist, but because cosmetic products are applied to the face, it's important that they be hygienic. Never buy a product in a package that has already been opened, or that seems less than clean. At home, store products carefully: Close packages after each use and don't keep them in a hot, steamy bathroom if you can help it.

Replace cosmetics at regular intervals. Here are some generally ac-

cepted guidelines on how long most cosmetics will stay fresh and free from bacterial contamination:

- *Liquid foundation* can be kept a maximum of a year and a half unopened, six months to one year after it's opened.
- *Face powder* can keep for up to three years unopened, but only one year after it's opened.
- *Powder blushers* can also stay fresh for about three years unopened, one year after they're opened.
- *Cream or gel blushes* can be kept two years unopened, but should be replaced within six months of opening the package.
- *Eye pencils* can be kept for one year unopened, for six months after opening.
- *Eye shadows* can be kept for one year unopened, for six months after opening.
- *Mascaras* can be kept for six months unopened, for three to six months after opening. (These are very conservative guidelines, I know, but mascara is especially vulnerable to contamination. Always discard all eye makeup products immediately if you develop any type of eye infection or irritation.)

In any case where the consistency, color, or odor of a makeup product has changed, it should be replaced—regardless of whether you've owned it for a single day or a year.

Practice safe makeup application. Use common sense when applying any makeup product: *Never* add saliva to a product to lighten its texture, and *never* share your makeup with anyone else. Don't use makeup on irritated or broken skin, or too close to the eyeball itself—and *never* apply cosmetics on the inside of either the upper or lower lid within the lash line. Makeup should not be applied while you're talking or distracted by other goings-on in the same room. This is especially true when you're applying eye makeup, which can be irritating at best and sometimes even dangerous if it gets inside the eyes. Never apply makeup anywhere near your eyes when sitting in a taxicab, train, plane, or car.

Invest in the best quality makeup tools—and keep them scrupulously clean. One of the secrets of a professional makeup artist is the tools he or she uses to give makeup a smooth, perfect finish. I recommend that any woman who wears makeup on an everyday basis make an investment in a quality set of makeup brushes made of natural materials—a good blusher brush, a loose-powder brush, and a lip brush at minimum (eye brushes are not a must, since cotton swabs can be used instead, and disposed of after every use for the ultimate in safety around the delicate eye area). It makes sense to invest, too, in a lesson from a makeup professional to learn the best ways to use these tools and how to care for them—usually a matter of cleansing the brushes in a gentle shampoo and letting them air-dry at least once a week. Failure to keep makeup tools clean is a commonly ignored source of skin problems, for makeup left on brushes collects bacteria from the air that is then introduced onto your skin, where it combines with skin oils to cause a reaction that may result in unsightly skin eruptions.

Always remove makeup before exercise and before going to sleep. It sounds so simple, but I can't tell you how many skin problems I have seen as a result of women who were "too tired" to cleanse their faces before going to bed at night—or who wanted to look their best for their exercise class. The most important safety advice I can give about makeup is that it should be removed before any activity that involves perspiration (even if it's just a vigorous walk around the block) or before going to sleep, a time when your skin needs to breathe and recuperate. Many women who can wear makeup without a problem develop skin reactions only when they wear makeup for too many hours at a time, so if you are just staying home for the evening, do your skin a favor and cleanse off your makeup as soon as you come home from work. In addition, if you have the time, try to cleanse off your makeup and apply fresh cosmetics before going out at night; our skin can collect dust and oils during the day, so applying "new" makeup over "old" to go out at night isn't the best idea. If you just have time for a touch-up, try to avoid putting on any additional oil-containing products and just touch up with a bit of powder eye shadow around eyes and powder blusher on the apple of your cheeks.

FOUNDATION
Perfect Skin Match

Choosing the right foundation depends on the same two important factors we've discussed before: your skin type and the color of your skin. Because foundation is the makeup that is worn closest to the skin, it must not be too oily (as it could encourage skin breakouts) nor contain too much alcohol (which could over-dry the complexion). Achieving a perfect color match with your skin is the key to avoiding the look of an artificial mask of makeup.

Choosing the Foundation That's Right for Your Skin Type. Read the ingredients found in the makeup, which are listed on the bottom of the bottle or the outside of the makeup package. If the formula contains mineral oil, it is fine for dry skin but too heavy for oily or combination skin. A woman with an oily complexion should choose a makeup with a matte finish, because this type of foundation will contain powder that will help to absorb excess skin oils. So-called pore-minimizing foundations are another good choice; they are usually powder-in-water emulsions that go on with a very matte finish and can be "buffed" down with a sponge to a smooth, natural-looking finish. Cream-formula or oil-in-water emulsion foundations are good choices for women with dry complexions, while oil-free, pancake, or matte foundations work well for combination skin.

Whatever type of foundation you choose, don't apply it directly to skin without the "buffer" layer of a lightweight moisturizer. Many women with oily skin hesitate to apply moisturizing lotions under their makeup because they think it gives skin a shiny look by midday. But you can easily tone down the shine with a dusting of loose translucent powder. Also, if your skin has any tendency at all to be sensitive, shielding your skin with this thin layer of moisturizer will reduce the chance of your developing a reaction caused by an ingredient in your foundation. One caveat: Choose a moisturizer that absorbs into the skin instantly and easily and that is matched to your skin type.

Choosing the Right Color of Foundation. Equally important to the way a foundation "wears" is that the shade is correctly matched to your skin color. Because it is not unusual for the skin of your face to be slightly lighter in color than the skin of your neck, most makeup experts recommend matching the shade of your makeup to the jawline. To do a fast shade test, apply a dot of foundation with a sponge or cotton swab to the skin near your jawline, then blend with your fingertip. Never test a foundation on the skin of your wrist or hand; if it matches your hands it may not match the skin of your face.

What do you do if you have a hard time finding a foundation that works for your skin color? Buy *two* foundations, one slightly lighter than your skin color, the other slightly darker, and blend them together in proportions that give you a perfect skin match. (It's best to buy both shades from the same company to get the best blending of color and formula.) If you have combination skin, you might want to buy the two shades in two different formulas—one for normal-to-dry skin, the other for normal-to-oily—to achieve the perfect skin texture as well as color match.

One final word on foundation color: Many women use foundation to try to change their skin color—for instance, to give the impression of a tan or of a porcelain-doll finish. While this may work for a photographer's model, or an actress on stage or in the movies, it won't work in everyday life, where a contrast between your artificial facial skin color and the skin of your arms, hands, or legs is more noticeable. For the most natural-looking, flattering result, stay as close to your natural skin tone as possible in choosing a foundation. The purpose of foundation is not to *change* your skin, but to give it smoother, more even texture and to produce a base for the rest of your makeup.

BLUSHER
A Touch of "Healthy" Color

Properly applied, blusher can give your face a healthy-looking glow. Choosing a blusher depends on your personal preference as well as an awareness of color, shading, and skin type.

Blushers come in four basic types:

Powder blushers are the most modern. They have a soft finish as well as the ability to produce as much or as little color as a woman desires. Powders work well on just about all skin types and should be the first choice for a woman who has oily or combination skin, since they will help to absorb excess skin oils without changing color. Powder blushers should be applied with a big, fluffy brush (the small brushes that are packaged with the blushers tend to produce a stripe of concentrated cheek color rather than a natural-looking result). Powder blushers should be applied over foundation or, if you have especially smooth skin and do not need foundation, can be applied simply over bare skin.

Cream blushers are suitable for normal-to-dry skin and camouflage fine lines or wrinkles better than powder blushers. Creams do tend to streak, though, so they must be applied carefully. For best results,

blend a bit of moisturizer into the blusher in the palm of your hand, then smooth onto cheeks using a moistened cosmetic sponge (it will give you more control of application than will using your fingertips). Apply blusher in a soft arc along the cheekbones, then blend the edges with your fingers or a soft sponge until there is no obvious line of demarcation where the blusher starts or ends. Never apply cream blusher in a circular motion—it will look very artificial.

Liquid blushers—or color rubs, as some companies call them—are sheer and can be used as either cheek color or an allover face tint. Liquid blushers are best used on normal or dry skin. For the most natural-looking results, blend a small amount of liquid blusher onto the skin with fingertips, working quickly for even coverage and a sheer finish.

Gel blushers are similar to liquids but more transparent; again, they work best on normal or dry skin. Because gels tend to streak, they must be applied gently with fingertips, then blended well to avoid obvious lines of demarcation. Gel blushers can be used as all over face color in the summertime when you don't want the additional coverage provided by foundation.

Choosing a blusher color is as important to the results (and the natural look of modern makeup) as is deciding on the type of formula to use. There are no hard and fast rules about color choices but, in general, choose a color that is complementary to your skin tone. Some tips in choosing a blusher color: *Fair-skinned blondes* might want to experiment with beige-pink and coral blushers, whereas *fair-skinned brunettes* often find rosy to pale pink shades flattering. *Olive-toned* complexions are complemented by reddish bronze, soft rose, or coral shades, whereas *black skin* can look great with a sheer hint of soft pink, pink-mauve, or blue-red blusher (avoid dark mauve blush as this tends to emphasize any ashiness in a complexion).

A final word on applying blusher: Make a V with your index and middle fingers, then place the V over your cheek with your fingertips, touching the top and bottom of the ear. Look in the mirror and you will get a general idea of where blusher should be applied. Avoid applying color too close to your nose, which can make it appear bigger, or too close to your eyes, which can take away from their beauty. Also keep in mind that blusher applied too high or too low on the cheeks can look unnatural. The best bet is to experiment—and always to blend blusher into the skin to avoid a painted-on look. And remember, it's easier to add more blusher than it is to take color away— so apply very little at first, blend, then check the results in the mirror before applying more.

EYE LIGHTING
Eye-Makeup Strategies

Our eyes are our most expressive features—and eye makeup can bring out the beauty of every woman's eyes. But proper application is key; applying too much eye makeup is something many women do, and the results are not at all flattering. Here are a dozen important tips on using makeup to make the most of your eyes:

1. Always apply eye makeup in a room with good lighting and a high-quality mirror—and not when you are in a hurry. Never apply eye makeup in a moving vehicle—be it car or train; a sudden jerk of the vehicle and you can poke yourself in the eye.

2. Apply eye makeup with a light hand—it is far easier to add more color than to subtract. Trying to rub away too much eye makeup can leave eyes looking red, teary, and *unattractive*.

3. Choose eye makeup formulas carefully. If you are sensitive to makeup products, problems are even more likely in the delicate eye area. Always store eye makeup properly and replace it promptly (see advice on makeup replacement on page 185).

4. If you use eye pencils, choose those with the softest tip for easier blending. Too much tugging or pulling at the skin around the eyes can lead to irritation in the short run, and can actually contribute to the formation of lines and wrinkles around your eyes in the long run.

5. Match your makeup to the time of day, your mood, your personal style. Today, many women prefer to use very soft, earthy colors in daytime makeup—and this goes for eye makeup as well. At night, adding a little more color, or a bit of shimmer around the eyes, is the only change needed.

6. For ease of application, begin your eye makeup with a concealer or a camouflage color under eyes, then apply eye shadow, and then eye-liner, if you want it. Finish with mascara.

7. Pay attention to your brows— but don't overtweeze or overshape them. The most modern look is to have neat but not unnaturally tweezed eyebrows with a full, not pencil-thin, shape. Experts recommend tweezing away only stray hairs under the brow, with the aim being

to have a neat shape, *not* to *re*shape the brow's natural arch or thickness. If in doubt, think of the type of brows that women such as model-actress Brooke Shields have—they are by no means obviously tweezed!

8. If you feel your eyebrows could use a little help, consult a professional. A makeup or skin care salon usually has someone on staff who, along with offering makeup lessons, can offer advice and help with brow grooming. If you are like many women who feel that, once you have an eyebrow tweezer in hand, you don't know when to stop, consider having your brows tweezed professionally. A makeup pro can also give you advice on using brow pencils for a natural, not made-up, look, to create the illusion of a somewhat thicker brow.

9. Opt for powder shadows, or soft powder pencils, rather than cream eye shadow for easier application and less chance of color "streaking" as the day or evening wears on. Powder shadows can provide a range of intensities depending on whether you apply with a moistened brush (for more intense, lasting color) or a dry one (for softer, more smudgeable color). Use a soft natural-bristle brush or a sponge-tipped applicator to apply powder shadow, and keep colors in the same color family, with darker colors to "shade" an area, lighter colors to highlight or emphasize (such as on the brow bone). While makeup professionals often use eye shadows to correct the shape of eyes or create the illusion of a somewhat differently shaped eye, this is very difficult for the average woman to do; shy away from the temptation to try to create changes in your appearance, unless you have had step-by-step personal-ized instruction from a makeup professional.

10. If you like liquid or cake eye liner, be aware that the results that you get may be old-fashionedly precise. The modern look of eye liner is a soft smudged line—which can be difficult to achieve with liquid or cake liner. The best bet is to use an angle-tipped brush and dilute liner by moistening the brush before you use it.

11. Don't overapply mascara. Always apply a single coat and allow it to dry for a few seconds before applying another coat—you may even find that you don't need the second coat at all. There is nothing less attractive than clumpy or spiky mascara, which often results from overuse rather than misuse of mascara. If you use a mascara with a built-in brush applicator, allow the mascara on the wand to air-dry a few seconds before applying it. If you find that your lashes still tend to stick together after you've applied mascara, try using a lash separator or lash comb—usually a metal comb (made of surgical steel or even gold) that can be used to comb through mascara after it's applied—and remove the excess. (*Note:* Clean your lash separator often with an alcohol-moistened cotton ball or it won't do its job very well.)

12. Use a cotton swab to clean up your eye makeup after it's applied. A moistened cotton swab can be used to "take down" too deep or too opaque eyeliner or shadow, or to blend together two different colors of shadow so there's no harsh line of separation.

LIP TRICKS
Color Plus

The modern way to apply lipstick is not to try to reshape your lips but to accent and emphasize the lip area. Trying to change your lips with color usually only produces a very artificial look.

The first step in applying lipstick is to prepare the lip surface—something that shouldn't be done only when you apply your makeup but should be part of a regimen of caring for the skin of your lips. Chapped lips not only look unattractive (and can sometimes hurt) but make it much more difficult to apply lipstick than when your lips are smooth and supple. I recommend always applying a moisturizing lip base (a colorless lip cream or, if you prefer, a commercial chapped-lip preparation or petroleum jelly) every day, even when you are not wearing lip color. As part of a facial in my salon, a lip moisturizer is always applied—a step many of my clients find surprising, but a step that emphasizes that skin care is a total concern, not merely targeted at one area of the face. Never apply lipstick directly to bare lips; the waxes in some lip colors can actually have a drying effect, so always buffer lip color with a moisturizing base. Whether or not you choose to use one of the new multipurpose lip bases—targeted at moisturizing plus holding color in place—is a matter of personal choice.

The most flattering way to apply lipstick is with a lip brush. Apply a thin coat of color, then dab a little gloss just in the center of lips. While color is a matter of personal choice, do be aware of the match between your skin tone and lipstick color: A too-orange lipstick, for example, is a very common makeup mistake and ends up giving the skin a pasty look. There's no need, today, to match your lipstick to your clothes, but you should choose a color that complements both your skin tone and the colors you are wearing.

SPECIAL NEEDS
Makeup Cover-Ups

While none of us feel that we have perfect complexions, for some women, there is a very real need for makeup as camouflage, as a way to deemphasize skin flaws, scars, or breakouts. Today, the good news is that there are several companies—Covermark, Dermablend, Clinique—that make products specially formulated to mask severe skin discoloration or scarring. Using these products requires special procedures, so discuss their use with an esthetician. Here are some basic starting points for corrective makeup use:

Cover-ups come in several different types of formulas. You will find coverage products in cream, powder, and stick formulas. While in the past, the thicker the product, the better it worked, today that is not always the case. Through use of opaque ingredients, such as titanium dioxide, companies are now making more "breathable" cover-up products. The key is to apply these products to skin that has been moisturized first, then to "seal" in the coverage by applying a dusting of translucent powder over the cream or stick cover-up.

Match all cosmetics, including skin-corrective products, to your skin color. The key to using corrective makeup is to blend any skin mark into the surrounding skin. The most natural-looking results come from using a cover-up product that is precisely matched to your skin color—and, of course, that will also

191

blend into your overall foundation. If you are using a skin-correcting formula only under your eyes, or on a birthmark on your cheek, always apply the coverage product under your foundation; then, once you apply a translucent foundation over it, it will seem as if your skin—rather than makeup—is what is showing through.

When covering scars, always discuss the safety of products with your dermatologist or surgeon first. After an accident or plastic surgery, the skin takes a period of weeks or months even to begin to heal; usually, there is a period of a week or two during which time it is advisable not to wear any cosmetic products at all. If you have any doubt about using makeup, don't. And don't overlook the important advice given to you by a doctor.

To cover dark circles, use as little cover-up as possible. One of the most common makeup mistakes that women make is to apply too much concealer under their eyes. The most effective results are actually achieved by applying concealer *under* the dark circles, since they are often caused by shadows cast by excess skin or fat pouches below the eyes. Always pat on small dots of concealer gently with fingertips, then blend upward into the darker area with feather-light strokes of your fingertips. Never use white undereye concealer; it looks totally unnatural and owl-like.

HYPOALLERGENIC
What Does It Mean?
❧

According to the American Academy of Dermatology, an estimated 6 percent of all allergic skin reactions can be traced to cosmetics—a number that is actually decreasing because of more thorough, sophisiticated testing of cosmetic products by manufacturers. Yet for many women, cosmetics that are labeled *hypo-allergenic, allergy-tested,* or *dermatologist-approved* appear to be safer than products that do not bear these labels. The surprising truth: Such labels are not regulated by the government and do not guarantee that a product underwent any more scrupulous testing than another, similar cosmetic.

The truth today is that just about every cosmetic, whether made by a large or small company, is put through a battery of tests before being put on sale; even "private label" products sold by small skin care salons are usually manufactured by much larger companies that do comprehensive premarket testing for safety and allergy. No company wants to manufacture a cosmetic that is likely to cause problems, and, today, the technology exists to determine whether a product is likely to cause a skin reaction in the majority of users. Still, the Food and Drug Administration—or any other government body—has not established a legal definition for terms such as *hypoallergenic*, so there is no way to determine by looking at a package what type of safety testing has actually been done. Similarly, while only a small percentage of products may be labeled *dermatologist-tested*, most testing of cosmetic safety is performed by dermatologists who work for private cosmetic-testing labs. And, experts emphasize, even in the most ideal conditions, the word *hypoallergenic* means least likely to cause an allergic reaction: In other words, in a small number of cases, such a product may in fact be the source of a skin allergy.

What is a woman with sensitive skin to do?

• Look for cosmetics that are labeled *fragrance-free*, because numerous studies by dermatologists have confirmed that fragrances in cosmetic formulations are the most common source of allergic reactions (one note of caution: Skip products that are labeled *unscented*, as these often contain masking fragrances that neutralize unpleasant odors of a product's raw ingredients).

• Choose products made by a manufacturer whose other cosmetics you have used in the past without a problem.

• If you have experienced a skin reaction in the past that was attributed to a specific ingredient such as lanolin or propylene glycol (two common cosmetic allergens), by all means read product labels to avoid that specific ingredient.

As a general rule, I tell all of my clients to be especially careful when using any type of cosmetic near the eyes. The eye area is the most vulnerable to cosmetic reactions because the skin is so thin and sensitive and because ingredients that never cause problems on the skin surface can be highly irritating if they happen to get inside the eye. If you suspect a problem has been caused by a cosmetic, bring the product, along with its package and ingredients label, to your dermatologist; through a new program cosponsored by the American Academy of Dermatology, any board-certified dermatologist can obtain help from most cosmetic companies in determining the ingredients list of specific cosmetic products.

SEASONAL SMARTS
Makeup Throughout the Year

At one time, makeup colors changed every season and women did actually go through a change in their look several times a year; today, most women have settled on a year-round look that they consider their personal style. Still, the fact remains that certain colors can be especially flattering at certain times of year. Here are some thoughts on making up for the seasons, some changes to consider and adapt to your own personal style:

Summer. This is the season for wearing less makeup, in terms of both texture and color. If your skin is in good condition, go without foundation this time of year, especially if you live in a climate that is humid as well as hot. If your job requires a more finished makeup, then at least go a bit lighter in texture in your makeup in summertime—or lighten the weight of your foundation by blending in a touch of cleansing lotion or astringent before applying it.

At this time of year, consider using cosmetics to "fake" a little bit of a tan (a drastic change looks obvious, as I said earlier), while keeping your skin protected with a makeup that contains sunscreen. (Or use a sunscreen in a moisturizer base in place of your usual moisturizer under your makeup.) Must-wear at this time of year: sunscreen on vulnerable skin areas such as around eyes, on cheekbones, and on lips. Rather than applying eyeshadow plus mascara—which can run in heat and humidity—consider going without eye

193

makeup during the day and simply using a soft brown eye crayon softly smudged around eyes at night. The only real makeup you'll need is a touch of soft pink blusher applied at "sunpoints" of the face—cheeks, temples, chin—to mimic the effect of a suntan.

Fall. This is a season of new beginnings, of a more polished approach to dressing than in summertime—and makeup usually looks a bit more "finished" too at this time of year. In fall, you'll probably want to wear makeup with slightly earthier tones, such as plums, khakis, greens, and grays around eyes, or rust tones on lips.

Translucent loose powder applied over makeup helps to set powders and allows makeup to last longer. For daytime, most women prefer a matte powder; if you like the look of a powder with a bit of shine, use it only at night and *sparingly*—for instance, just on cheeks—not all over the face.

Because the weather gets a bit cooler and the air a bit drier at this time of year, remember the importance of applying moisturizer under your makeup, not only to give your makeup a smoother finish but to protect skin as well. It's a good idea to apply moisturizer, then wait a minute or two for it to be absorbed into skin, before applying your makeup. If your skin has a tendency to be oily, choose a lightweight lotion-formula moisturizer and a foundation formulated specifically for oily complexions. Women with dry skin should use a richer moisturizer and a foundation that also contains moisturizing ingredients.

Winter. This season usually marks a continuation of fall colors but with one important concern: that all make-up formulas help to safeguard skin moisture during this driest time of year. Never apply makeup without applying moisturizing lotion first, and consider a switch to a creamier foundation and cream blushers. Always apply a base of eye cream around eyes before putting on color—and don't overlook eyelashes, which can also dry out and break in wintertime, especially if you wear mascara every day. Switch to creamier lipsticks that contain moisturizing ingredients plus sunblock if you aren't already using such formulas.

Spring. In this season, makeup colors are often softer, slightly pinker, more romantic in tone, and the texture can also be somewhat lighter than you wear in wintertime. If your skin tends to be oily, this is the time of year to go for more powder-based products and few creams, to help absorb skin oils and prevent breakouts. Women with dry skin will want to be sure to apply a richer moisturizer under their makeup and to wait a few minutes to allow the moisturizer to be absorbed before putting on any cosmetics.

Because spring is a season when we feel like spending more time outdoors, it's also important to think in terms of makeup as protection—and to look for cosmetics that contain sunscreening and moisturizing ingredients. Another option is to use a moisturizer-based sunscreen product instead of your usual moisturizer as an undermakeup base.

Part of the attractiveness of springtime, too, is the move to softer colors; take inspiration from the palette of nature around you for your makeup, considering a move to soft pinks, pale golden tones, and clear reds (if your skin can take them). The only rule is to keep your makeup in complementary tones—and to use strong color only on a single feature (if at all) to avoid an overly made-up look. A bright pink lipstick, for example, is especially attractive when you keep your eye makeup and cheek color minimal, while a green eye crayon can add a bit of unexpected color when you keep cheeks and lips very toned down.

16

Travel Bound
– Women
on the Go

Today, the numbers of women who travel—for business and pleasure—is on the rise. We are frequent flyers, train-takers, and drivers—and the change of climate that can be wonderful for our spirits or our souls can pose unexpected hazards for our complexions. It's no secret that our skin changes from one season to the next, but have you ever thought about the "instant season switch" effected by a one-and-a-half–hour plane trip from the breezy fall temperatures of New York to the still hot, humid atmosphere of Miami? Changes in local water, temperature, humidity, lack of sleep, and jet lag can all take their toll on your skin—unless, of course, you prepare for these changes. In this chapter, I'll give you a world traveler's guide to great-looking skin, and tell you the secrets that women who travel for a living (models, actresses, flight attendants)—and whose livelihoods depend on their looking good in every time zone, climate, and time of day—have come to rely on.

PREP TIME
What to Do Before You Go

As you prepare for your trip, whether it's around the country or around the world, take a few minutes to think about your skin—what your needs are at home and what they are likely to be wherever you're headed. While it's a good idea to have certain skin treatments done ahead of time— for instance, to have a facial at home rather than in a strange country—you don't want to schedule the appointment for the morning of your departure, when nervous tension can increase your skin's sensitivity to usually benign treatments. Here is a pretravel plan for common beauty treatments:

Skin-Caring. Don't try a brand-new skin care regime before you leave town. If it doesn't "agree" with your skin, you won't want to hit the road with a rash, allergy, or acne breakout. Instead, stick to your tried and true cleansers, moisturizers, and makeups. Save any new products for when you're at home, so if you do have a problem, you can consult a skin care pro or dermatologist right away. Changes in climate (especially exposure to sun or wind) can make skin much more sensitive to certain harsh ingredients in skin care products, such as alcohol, preservatives, or fragrance, so it's best not to embark on a new program when you know you'll be heading south to the tropics in another week's time.

Facials. If you possibly can, schedule your regular facial a week or so before your trip; that way, you'll start out with your skin as thoroughly cleansed as possible, and minimize the chances of developing excessive skin dryness or breakouts while you're away. Your facialist can also advise you about any special products you should bring along with you, depending on the climate you are headed for. If you are going to a dry, hot climate, for example, you might need to bring some richer moisturizers along with sunscreen; if you're headed for heat and humidity, you might need a "lightening" of your usual skin care routine (more on this later).

Manicures and Pedicures. These are key to a neat, groomed appearance during travel. Always have a professional manicure a day before you go away (especially on a business trip, where the first thing you will probably do is shake your client's hand, and you don't want him or her to notice your chipped red fingernails before hearing your business presentation). If you're going to a warm weather climate where you'll be wearing sandals or going barefoot at the pool or beach, by all means have a pedicure to remove calluses and dry skin and to groom and shape your toenails. If you want to have a manicure while you're away, bring a bottle of your favorite nail polish along with you; the last thing you'll want is to end up in a beauty salon in a strange city in which the only color nail polish available is burgundy or navy blue!

Waxing. This should always be done at least two days before you go away—and should never be done for the first time before you are going out of town. If you have waxing done regularly, you know that it can leave skin sensitive for a day or so afterward—and can particularly increase your sensitivity to swimming in salt or chlorine water. I advise my clients who have regular leg and bikini-area waxings to come in three days before they are planning a trip, to minimize any chances of adverse skin reactions.

Electrolysis. These treatments should always be done at least two weeks in advance of a trip, to minimize the chances of reactions caused by traveling to another climate. Properly done, electrolysis should not cause scars or severe reactions, but it can cause skin to be a bit more sensitive than usual and can also leave *slight* redness or irritation on highly delicate skin. Never start electrolysis right before you're going away;

because the treatments need to be properly timed, you'll want to work out a thorough schedule of treatments with your practitioner.

Hair Conditioning. This treatment should be thought of as pretrip insurance that your hair will behave while you're out of town. The last thing any woman wants, after all, is to waste time on a business trip *or* vacation fussing with her hair. A super salon-conditioning treatment makes particular sense if you'll be heading to a spot where you're likely to be outdoors a great deal or swimming in either salt or chlorine water, as outdoor activities and swimming can be particularly drying to every type of hair, especially if you color or perm yours.

AIRPLANE AIR
Skin and Hair Hazard
≈≈

The most common complaints I get from my clients who travel a great deal is the effect that frequent airplane trips can have on their skin and their hair. If you have a dry complexion, both the lack of fresh air and the low humidity of an airplane cabin can greatly increase skin flakiness, dryness, and irritation. Women with oily complexions often complain that they develop dry patches of skin on cheeks and chin during plane travel, then have a "rebound" of excessive oiliness and breakouts later on. Simply put, the environment of an airplane is not kind to a woman's complexion or her hair, regardless of age or skin or hair type.

What to do: Arm yourself ahead of time. If you possibly can, don't wear makeup while you travel; instead, apply a rich moisturizer to skin the morning of your flight and reapply it during any plane trip longer than one or two hours. Don't forget to wear eye cream as well—the delicate skin around your eyes is particularly prone to dryness and irritation. If you must wear makeup while you travel, always make it water-based (foundation and undermakeup primer or moisturizer).

Never drink alcohol on a plane. Alcohol—and caffeine—are natural diuretics, robbing your body of fluids and minimizing the amount of moisture available to skin cells. The result of alcohol or caffeine intake plus airplane air is taut, dry skin that is much more likely to become sensitive to ingredients in makeup or moisturizers.

Carry a spritzer of mineral water with you on a plane and use it to refresh and moisturize your complexion (if you're too embarrassed to do this while sitting in your seat, simply make a quick trip to the bathroom).

Always wear a lip balm or moisturizing lip color on board a plane to prevent lips from drying or cracking.

Carry a minitube of hand cream in your purse or carry-on bag and reapply it several times during your flight, especially if you wash your hands while on board the plane. If you're wearing short sleeves, apply the cream to arms and elbows also.

If dry airplane air causes eye irritations, apply cotton pads soaked in distilled water or cool milk (the flight attendant will happily oblige) to closed lids for several minutes. This should provide some soothing relief. (If you wear contact lenses, consider wearing your glasses instead to avoid unnecessary eye discomfort.)

Finally, a few minutes before the prelanding seat belt sign comes on, go to the ladies room and cleanse your face, then apply a moisturizer, water-based foundation, a bit of mas-

cara, powder blusher, and lip gloss. This way, anyone who is meeting you will think you look wonderfully fresh after such a long flight—and you will have protected your skin from any adverse reactions of plane travel.

Note: The same basic guidelines apply if you're taking a long train or car trip, as any static period of time in a closed environment is likely to rob skin of moisture.

CLIMATE CONTROL
Travel Factors

The basic premise of skin caring during travel is that any change of climate, food, and water will most certainly affect your skin. How you care for your skin, however, will determine the extent of travel's impact.

Hot, Dry Climates. If you're heading to a place with lots of heat and little humidity, pack plenty of sunscreen in a nonalcohol base, and rich body and face moisturizing creams and lotions to protect your skin and minimize dryness and flakiness. When swimming, always apply a rich moisturizing cream to your face and body, over your usual sunscreen, to seal in skin moisture and protection. Keep your skin lubricated at all times—applying two layers of moisturizer to face and body after a bath or shower. Don't forget to cleanse your face gently, and always to apply eye cream under makeup.

Hot and Humid Climates. For tropical places, what you'll want are the lightest, most protective skin products you can find—for instance, lightweight, nonclogging sunscreen formulas, sheer but protective moisture lotions, lip balm with sunscreen, and a lightweight eye cream. Be aware that you'll need to cleanse your face more often, but that you'll want to be as gentle as possible to prevent irritation. Since humidity increases oil production, you might want to pack a toner or astringent (without alcohol if your skin is naturally dry) to use in the morning, at midday, and at bedtime. Never use oil-based makeup in this type of climate; switch to a water-based foundation, and powdered eye and cheek colors instead of cream-based ones.

Cold, Dry Climates. Wintery areas will present you with a real challenge, since both the cold temperature and lack of humidity rob skin of the moisture that keeps it looking smooth and young. If you also have a problem with broken capillaries as well as dry and flaky skin, don't overtreat your skin.

Do avoid soap, however, whatever your skin type. Wash your face with a mild cleansing lotion to soften the skin and slough off dead surface cells. Rinse repeatedly with lukewarm—not hot—water.

If your skin is normal-to-dry, wear an oil-based foundation for additional protection (a water-based makeup will allow too much moisture to evaporate off skin's surface, increasing its susceptibility to flaking). Also try a cream or gel blusher instead of powder, then finish your makeup—as always—with translucent powder.

Keep your lips lubricated at all times to prevent chapping and cracking. Under lipstick, apply a clear lip balm or cream; if you're skipping lip color, don't skip protection. If you'll be in the sun—even when the temperatures are low—use an SPF 15 lip protectant.

Be aware that long, hot baths can dehydrate the skin; instead, take a quick shower or bathe in lukewarm water. After toweling off gently, slather a luxurious body lotion or cream from head to toe, while skin is still damp. Reapply body moisturizer before bedtime.

Watch out for scaly skin on elbows, knees, and shoulders in cold weather. Extra moisturizing in these vulnerable skin areas is a must—use a product with a petrolatum base.

Avoid misting your face with mineral water in cold weather. And never go outside when skin is still damp.

In this and any climate drink plenty of fluids (especially water) to moisturize your skin from the inside out. Again, avoid drinking too much alcohol or caffeine, as these are both natural diuretics.

SKIN SAVVY
*Trying Out Beauty Services
on the Road*

Many of my clients who travel a great deal tell me horror stories of getting a haircut in a foreign city only to find that their once-classic look had gone avant-garde—or, worse yet, punk. Obviously, there are certain services that you can try out in a strange city or foreign country, and others you should avoid.

I always try to schedule a *massage* when I am traveling for business. The tension of tightly packed business appointments conducted after a less than perfect night's sleep always puts me in need of a good rubdown. This is also usually a service that is danger-free; by inquiring of the concierge in my hotel as to which beauty salons nearby offer a Swedish massage, I have never had a bad experience yet. (One thing never to do, of course, is simply to pick a masseuse out of a phone book; always get a recommendation.)

The only time I suggest having a *facial* away from home is if you are going to a "branch" of a salon you regularly visit at home, or have had a recommendation from your usual facialist. Unfortunately, the reality is that many people who call themselves skin care experts are lacking in proper training and standards; the last thing you'll want to do is suffer the scars of an overzealous skin cleansing, or find that you have had an adverse reaction to a new cream. Likewise, don't attempt a "self-facial" while on the road; picking at your skin causes redness and irritation in the short run and can lead to permanent scarring in the long run. If you have a tendency to break out, ask your dermatologist or skin care expert for advice on what type of "emergency skin formula" to bring with you.

If you want to get a *haircut* in a salon that you are not familiar with, you are undoubtedly taking a risk that you won't like the results. Better to ask for a slight trim than to go for a total restyling—and best of all to go simply for a luxurious conditioning treatment, "comb-out," or evening style rather than a haircut.

The one exception to this advice is when you are spending your vacation at a top-quality health spa. The best spas around the world aim to be total beauty and health resorts—and there you will find facials, masseuses, manicurists, and hairstylists who have the highest standards of training and expertise. To get the most out of your stay, try all of the services offered at least once.

FOOD SAVVY—STAYING HEALTHY WHEN YOU TRAVEL

We're all familiar with stories of Mexican vacations ruined by the untoward effects of strange waters on a traveler's body—or of illness in a foreign country due to overindulging in food and wine. A little-known fact: Unusual eating patterns during travel can also have a negative effect on your skin's appearance.

To prevent sudden flushing of your complexion, or a rash due to an unexpected food allergy, try to stick to those foods you usually eat at home. An occasional, selective taste of local specialties is fine—but don't subject your body to an onslaught of unfamiliar spices and foods. (Staying away from a constant intake of hot, spicy food is especially important for women who have sensitive skin, as their complexions often flush easily.)

Peeled fresh fruits and vegetables are always a sensible choice because of their high water content, which the body needs to maintain healthy, supple skin.

Whenever possible, choose broiled fish, poultry, or veal for their low fat content; stay away from a constant intake of heavy cream sauces. Not only are heavy foods unhealthy in terms of their high fat content; they also can lead to indigestion—and no one looks or feels attractive with an upset stomach. Be aware that salty foods can cause water retention in your face as well as your body—this is the reason many women complain to me that, during travel, they feel as if they have constant bags under their eyes. Drink sodium-free mineral water whenever possible to help "flush out" your system; fresh fruit juices are another smart choice.

One thing that I do whenever I travel is to pack a supply of multiple-vitamin pills as nutritional insurance for those times that I can't manage to eat the balanced diet that I try to get at home.

TRAVEL SMARTS
What to Take Along

Any woman who travels often knows that it makes sense to travel light. As far as your grooming kit goes, here's what I recommend as the most minimal but complete list of supplies.

- Mild liquid or cream cleanser
- Cotton balls or pads (never use tissues on skin; they can be too harsh, especially on sensitive skin)
- Light and heavy moisturizer (use the light one daily, the heavy one when you're in the sun or cold, or as a night cream if you need one)
- Light, nongreasy eye cream
- Hand and body lotion
- Gentle mask (applying and rinsing off a mask takes just five minutes in your hotel room and can restore your energy and your skin)
- Sunscreen (SPF 15 a must)
- Herbal water or Evian mist (optional)
- Water-based foundation
- Translucent loose powder
- Two cosmetics brushes—a large one for powder and a small one for blusher
- Mascara (black or brown)
- Lip gloss
- Creamy lipstick
- Blusher (powder or cream)
- Disposable makeup sponges
- Gray or soft brown eye shadow or eye pencil

With this basic list, you'll have all the skin caring and makeup you'll need for day or night, summer or winter travel. Of course, you may want to add a particular product if it's a special favorite—such as a shimmery powder for black-tie evening makeup, or a bronzer in place of foundation.

MAKEUP ON THE RUN

One thing I have learned from my travels is that you never have time between appointments. Somehow, with late planes or traffic jams, the free time on your schedule inevitably evaporates. One thing that is essential to looking well-groomed and polished is being able to apply your makeup quickly, so you can sleep a few extra minutes in the morning (which heaven knows you'll need) and can go quickly from day to evening with a few minutes to shower, apply makeup, and change your clothes.

My basic makeup plan: Apply foundation (preferably water-based unless you're in a particularly cold, dry climate) with a disposable sponge. Use a dark gray or soft brown pencil to line eyes very close to lashes; smudge with a cotton swab or soft, small-angled makeup brush. Apply brown or black mascara. Use a soft natural-bristle brush to apply powder blusher to tips of cheekbones, chin, and edges of forehead (where the sun would strike your skin). Then apply a bit of matte lip color and, finally, loose translucent powder with an oversize natural-bristle brush. All the time that's needed is three to five minutes maximum. And the look is as polished, as neat, as when you spend twenty minutes or more applying an endless number of products. Besides, it's much more stylish to wear less makeup, less color.

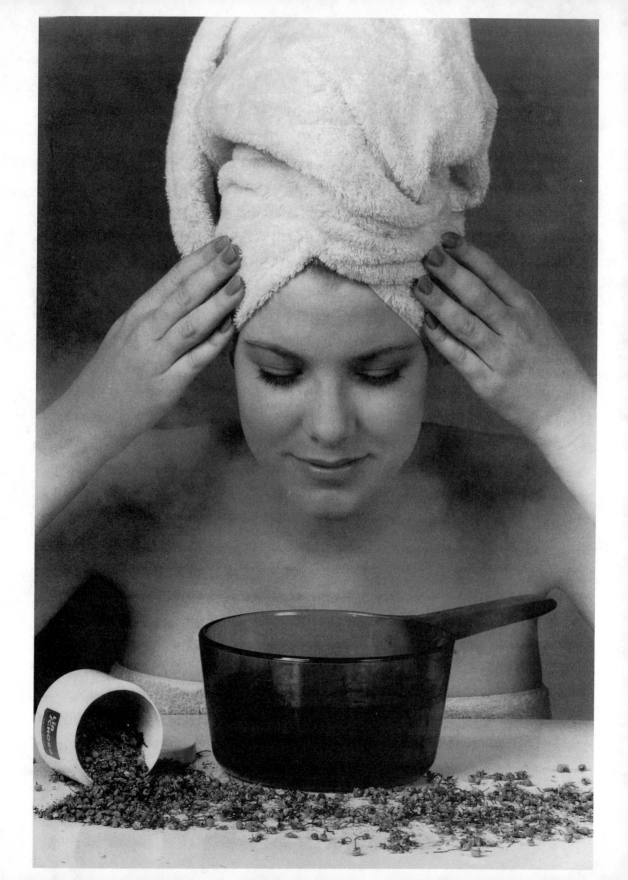

17

Make-it-Yourself
Skin Care

One of the most common question I am asked by women is whether natural or homemade skin care products are better for their skin than the store-bought variety. While the most important factor is to use products that are geared to your skin type, it is my opinion that many homemade skin cleansers and tonics do add to the pleasure of taking care of your skin, and can also help the results. While they may not be better, they are a pleasant alternative. Here, then, is my selection of skin care recipes to use at home, many of them based on generations-old ideas from Europe and Israel. (*Note:* All home recipes should be stored in the refrigerator and can be kept for up to two weeks unless otherwise noted. Never leave these products out at room temperature for longer than it takes to use them.)

GENTLE SKIN CLEANSERS

The following recipes should be used on the face only:

Cucumber Milk Cleanser (for dry skin)
Use a blender to liquify 1 cucumber; strain to remove seeds. Mix together equal amounts of cucumber juice and whole milk. Apply to skin with cotton ball and rinse immediately with cool water several times. (Can be stored in the refrigerator and used over the course of one week.)

Vitamin Cleanser
(for normal-to-oily skin)
Soak 1 cup of dried kidney beans overnight. The next day, drain and add enough water to cover the beans, and simmer for 2 hours. Strain, retaining the liquid to use as a cleanser. Apply with a cotton ball;

rinse immediately with cool, clear water. (Can be stored in the refrigerator and used for one week.)

Almond Milk Cleansing Lotion
(for oily skin)
Put ¼ cup almonds into food processor and process into almond meal. Blend together almond meal, ¾ cups rosewater, and 1 tablespoon witch hazel. Apply to skin with cotton ball; rinse immediately with cool water.

Sweet Butter Cleansing Cream
(for sensitive skin/pregnant women)
Soften 2 tablespoons sweet (salt-free) butter; mix in a glass bowl with 4 tablespoons mineral oil and 2 tablespoons sesame oil. Add 1 tablespoon distilled water and spoon into a wide-mouthed jar. Smooth mixture onto face with fingertips; massage into skin with gentle circular massage for one minute. Rinse with warm water several times. (Store in refrigerator; soften at room temperature for a few minutes before use; discard after 1 week.)

MOST EFFECTIVE MOISTURIZERS

As with store-bought moisturizers, these masks should all be applied to clean bare skin with fingertips. They are intended for the face and can be worn under makeup or alone.

Sensitive-Skin Moisturizer
(also can be used by new mothers)
Warm 3 teaspoons honey in a double boiler. Remove from the heat and slowly add ½ cup almond oil and ½ cup avocado oil (available in health food stores or supermarkets). Drop by drop, stir in 3 teaspoons rosewater. (Keep refrigerated for one day before use; discard after two weeks.)

Superrich Moisture Cream
(for very dry skin; can double
as night cream)

Mix 1 tablespoon olive oil with 1 tablespoon corn oil and 1 teaspoon almond oil; mix in 2 teaspoons water. Spoon into wide-mouthed jar. (Store in refrigerator and allow to soften at room temperature for a few minutes before using.)

Honey Night Cream
(for all skin types)

Whip the yolk of 1 egg and slowly add 10 drops of almond oil and 2 tablespoons of honey. Continue to whip the mixture until creamy; store in wide-mouthed jar.

SKIN TONERS AND
ASTRINGENTS

These recipes should be applied to skin after cleansing and can be left on or rinsed off, depending on what you prefer.

Dill Astringent Lotion
(for all skin types)

Boil 1 cup fresh dill in 2 cups spring water. Allow to cool; filter through a fine piece of cheesecloth. Apply to skin after cleansing with a soft cotton ball.

Orange Cleanser
(for all skin types)

Put 1 slice orange, 1 slice lemon, 1 tablespoon sugar, and 1 cup of milk into a saucepan and heat over low flame. Cool and put into refrigerator. Use as postcleansing skin freshener.

Blueberry Tonic
(for normal-to-oily skin)

Mix together 3 tablespoons stemmed, crushed blueberries and ½ cup sour cream or plain yogurt. Apply to face
and neck and rinse off after a few minutes with tepid water.

Red Wine Rejuvenator
(for combination and oily skin)

Mix ½ cup red wine (or apple juice), 2 tablespoons distilled water and 2 tablespoons cold chamomile tea. Apply to just-cleansed face with clean cotton ball. Follow with lukewarm-water rinse.

NATURAL MÉLANGE
MASKS

Grape Mask (for dry skin)

In a blender, blend 1 cup seedless grapes (red or green) until pulpy. Apply to face and neck before showering; leave on no more than 5 minutes; rinse off in shower with warm-water splashes. (This is a perfect once-a-week reviver for dry skin.)

Egg White Mask
(for oily/combination skin)

Beat the whites of 2 eggs with some fresh, finely minced yarrow and sage (available from stores that sell fresh herbs). When the mixture forms peaks, apply to clean skin. Leave on for 15 minutes, then rinse off with warm-water splashes. Follow with an application of a moisturizer geared to your skin type.

Papaya Mask
(for blotchy/blackhead-prone skin)

Mash 1 papaya; apply to clean skin. Leave on for 10 minutes; rinse with warm-water splashes.

Banana Mask
(for normal-to-dry skin)

Mash ½ banana. Add 1 tablespoon honey and 2 tablespoons sour cream. Blend well, then apply to clean skin.

Leave on for 10 minutes, then rinse with lukewarm water. Follow with a rich moisturizer.

Avocado Mask (for all skin types)

Mash 2 tablespoons avocado; blend with 1 tablespoon honey and 2 drops lemon juice. Apply to clean skin; leave on for 10 minutes. Rinse off with lukewarm water.

BODY BOOSTERS
Skin Treats for Back, Chest, Arms, and Hands

Strawberry Mask
(for all skin types)

Mash 15 fresh strawberries with 1 cup sour cream. Apply to skin with cotton balls dipped in lukewarm water. Leave on for 10 minutes; rinse off in shower or bath.

Clay Mask
(for oily/problem-prone skin)

Add 2 tablespoons mineral water to 3 tablespoons fuller's earth (a clay-like substance sold in drugstores). Blend in 1 tablespoon carrot juice. If needed, add a pinch more fuller's earth to create a soft clay. Apply to back, chest, or arms; leave on for 15 minutes. Rinse off with warm water in the shower.

Lavender Soak
(for all skin types)

To add to the bath: Mix together 2 tablespoons lavender flowers, 3 tablespoons bay leaves, 4 tablespoons fine oatmeal, and 4 tablespoons bran. Simmer with enough water to cover for 1 hour. Strain through cheesecloth. Add liquid to warm bath water.

Skin-Softening Lotion
(for all skin types)

Peel one 3/4-pound cucumber and liquefy in a blender or food processor; strain and retain the juice. Barely warm 1/4 cup chamomile tea; add the cucumber juice and 2 tablespoons glycerine, stirring well. Bottle when cool and refrigerate. Apply to skin after a bath or shower; do not rinse.

Hand Smoother

Mix a few drops of glycerine with a few drops of lemon oil. Massage into your hands before going to sleep.

Skin-Nourishing Body Oil

Before a bath, rub vitamin E or olive oil into dry skin areas—feet, knees, elbows, arms, and tops of shoulders. As the bathwater runs, spend a few minutes in the steamy environment of the bathroom to help the oil penetrate into the skin. Do not add additional oils to the bathwater—the warmth of the water will further encourage the oil on your skin to penetrate flaky skin layers. Cleanse your skin and pat dry; follow up with a rich body lotion.

HAIR HELPERS

Egg and Oil Conditioner
(for weak, brittle hair)

Apply 2 tablespoons of olive oil to scalp and massage lightly. Beat the yolk of 1 egg in a small bowl and apply it to hair, working from ends up to, but not into, scalp. Put on a plastic shower cap and go into the shower. After cleansing your face and body, remove the shower cap and shampoo as usual. Hair should feel softer and have more body. (If your hair is very *dry or weak, repeat this treatment as often as once a week.)*

Last Rinse

One of my favorite ways to use herbs is to make a "tea" to use as a final hair rinse (after it's thoroughly cooled, of course). Here, what works for different hair types: Chamomile *can help to soften and subtly lighten* blond hair; marigold leaves *(sometimes sold as* calendula) *can also help to give blond hair back some of its natural shine;* rosemary *lends luster and sheen to brown hair;* sage *helps to soften and condition dry hair;* lemon verbena *helps return the hair to a healthy pH; and* elderberries *help bring out the "blue" in dark black hair.*

Index

Caffeine, 200
Calamine powder mask, 42
Calcium, 157, 158
Capillaries, broken, 42–43
Chamomile, in shampoo, 106
Chamomile tea compresses, 179
Chanel, Coco, 2
Chapped hands, 56, 169
Chapped lips, 52, 56, 191
Chest
  blemishes on, 130
  sunburn of, 8
Chlorine, effect of, 15, 168
Cleansers, applying, 28
Cleansing creams, natural milk in,
  64
Cleansing skin, 42
  educating children about, 77
  of entire body, 13
Cleopatra, 132
Clay, in masks, 64, 79
Clogged pores, 11
Clothing, washing, 131
Cocoa butter, in skin products,
  65
"Cold creams," xvi
Collagen, 4, 89
Colors, flattering to skin, 51–52
Complexion
  smoothness of, 30
  swimming as aid to, 24
  in teens, 51
  in twenties, 51
Conditioners, 17, 32, 48, 109
  home recipes for, 110–111
Conditioning
  before traveling, 199
  in winter, 45
Cornstarch, 76
Cosmetics, sensitivity to, 42
Cream blushers, 188
Cream foundations, 70
Crow's feet, 81
Cryosurgery, 9
Cucumber, in skin products,
  65
Cuticles, 143, 144, 147

Dandruff, 46
Deep peeling treatments, 29–30
  recommendation against, 30
Dehydration, 8
Deodorants, difference between
  antiperspirants and, 12
Depilatories, 117–118
Dermabrasion, 29
Dermis, 89
Diet, 154–161
  balanced diet, 154–155
  breakfast, 159
  complex carbohydrates, 156
  crash diets, 161
  desserts, 160
  diet-skin connection, 78
  eating more than once a day, 155
  fat and cholesterol, avoiding, 155
  fiber in, 155–156
  food cravings, 160
  overeating, avoiding, 155
  salt, avoiding, 156
  substituting herbs and spices for
    salt, 159–160
  sugar, avoiding, 156
  travel and, 202–203
Dry scalp, 31–32
  in winter, 46
Dry skin, 60, 96
  dry houses as cause of, 36
  in summer, 23
    cleansing, 12
    sun and, 2
  in winter, 43

Eccrine glands, 11
Eczema, 89
Elastin, 4, 89
Electroysis, 118–119
  for hair around nipples, 137
  before traveling, 199
Emollients, 55
Epidermis, 88
Estrogen, 89
Europe, luxury spas in, 99

211

About the Authors

LIA SCHORR

No list of the top skincare experts in the country is complete without her name. She has appeared on the "Oprah Winfrey Show," "Phil Donahue," "The Today Show," Cable Health Network, and news shows in New York City, Los Angeles, and Chicago. Her advice has been featured in magazines including *Town and Country, Vogue, Harper's Bazaar, Mademoiselle, Self, American Health, Prevention, Elle, McCall's, Ladies' Home Journal, W, Working Woman,* and *Redbook*. She's been interviewed by *USA Today*, Eastern Airlines and Pan Am magazines, and in publications in Israel, Japan, Brazil, England, and Italy. She has been a regular columnist in publications including *Big Beautiful Woman, Today's Living, Better Health and Living, Beauty Handbook,* and *Better Nutrition*, and was recently named a contributing editor of the *National Beauty School Journal*. A member of Cosmetic Executive Women and the Society of Cosmetic Chemists, Ms. Schorr has lectured to organizations literally all over the world.

For the past seven years, Lia Schorr has had her own skin care salon in New York City, where she has tended to the complexions of some of the most famous women—and men—in the world. She recently introduced a new line of skin care products called Bio Botanics Skincare for Women that is sold through the salon and by mail. She is the author of *Lia Schorr's Skin Care Guide for Men*, also published by Prentice Hall Press.

SHARI MILLER SIMS

Currently Senior Health Director of *Self* magazine, Shari Miller Sims has over a decade of experience writing and editing about beauty and health for major magazines. A former Beauty and Health Writer for *Vogue* and Associate Editor of *McCall's*, she is also the coauthor of *Lia Schorr's Skin Care Guide for Men*.